The Little Qanun of Ibn Sina

Kadircan H. Keskinbora

The Little Qanun of Ibn Sina

Little Model of the Great Qanun

PETER LANG

Bibliographic Information published by the Deutsche Nationalbibliothek
The Deutsche Nationalbibliothek lists this publication in the Deutsche Nationalbibliografie; detailed bibliographic data is available online at http://dnb.d-nb.de.

Library of Congress Cataloging-in-Publication Data
A CIP catalog record for this book has been applied for at the Library of Congress.

Turkish edition: İbn Sina'nın Küçük Tıp Kanunu Ciltli / The Little Canon (or Qanun) of Ibn Sina
Istanbul: Bahcesehir Universitesi, 2015

The views expressed in this book are purely that of the author himself and may not in any circumstances be regarded as stating an official position of Bahçeşehir University

ISBN 978-3-631-79476-0 (Print)
E-ISBN 978-3-631-80324-0 (E-PDF)
E-ISBN 978-3-631-80325-7 (EPUB)
E-ISBN 978-3-631-80326-4 (MOBI)
DOI 10.3726/b16195

Peter Lang – Berlin · Bern · Bruxelles · New York · Oxford · Warszawa · Wien

This publication has been peer reviewed.

www.peterlang.com

There are some prescriptions given in this book, which have been translated exactly as they were written 1,000 years ago, including the ingredients mentioned. Under no circumstances should readers today take these as medical advice. Authorized physicians should be consulted for any treatment.

Foreword

Although very few copies of the Qanun-u Saghir (Little Qanun of Ibn Sina), Avicenna's world renowned Canon of Medicine exist today, the Handwritten Works libraries in Istanbul, Turkey remain one of the wealthiest sources of such works. There are four copies of this particular work in Turkey:

1. SÜLEYMANİYE Library REIS-UL-KUTTAB Collection Nb.103
2. SÜLEYMANİYE Library FATİH Collection Nb.3593
3. BAYAZIT Library UMUMİ Collection Nb.4123
4. BAYAZIT Library VELİYÜDDİN EFENDİ Collection Nb.2529

During the course of this work, four of the copies have been carefully read, revealing no differences apart from the prayers and identification information included at the end by the scribes; meaning that these four copies are identical in terms of style, wording and outline.

This book has been translated from the 2529 numbered book in the VELİYÜDDİN EFENDİ Collection at the BAYAZIT Library into Turkish. The international scientific community has been informed of the existence of this translation numerous times through presentations at international conferences. It was subsequently translated into English, and presented to scientists on various occasions for their perusal. Scientists working in this area have been aware of this work for nearly 6 years.

To answer a question commonly posed by scientists as to whether this book is a "Kanunçe-Kanunche (Canon summary)":

Not only could a Kanunçe be a 'special booklet' written by any scientist making references to Avicenna's Canon, it could also be a 'review/contribution booklet' written by a scientist and include critical views, contributions or additions to one of more topics in the Canon. Therefore, the size, language, style, wording and section divisions vary from booklet to booklet.

However, in the Qanun-u Saghir, the size of the books vary only by a few pages due to the nature of the handwriting, but are identical in terms of language, sections, content and so on.

The Qanun-u Saghir is a book comprising ten articles and 100 topics. The scribes who produced the copies have also stated that it was written by Ibn Sina (Avicenna). It consists of individual articles focusing on the creation of the human, the body, followed by a systematic description of the human body from head to toe, based on the medical scientific classifications.

This new edition of Ibn Sina's Little Qanun has been printed by Peter Lang Co. My previous translation has been re-edited meticulously and peer-reviewed. I want to thank everyone involved in the process at the company for their invaluable contribution.

Little Qanun of Ibn Sina like any printed book, this one may contain various errors, for which I apologize to the reader in advance and thank them for their understanding. For comments, contributions and thoughts, please do not hesitate to write to:

hidirkadircan.keskinbora@med.bau.edu.tr; kadircan.keskinbora@gmail.com

With my sincere hope that this book contributes to science and humanity, I remain

Kadircan H. KESKİNBORA, MD, Ph.D

Foreword (for Bahçeşehir Univ. edition)

Ibn Sina wrote many books on various scientific branches such as philosophy, religion, music, medicine, astronomy, physics, and natural sciences. Some sources state that the number of the books he has written is over 240; 153 of these have been found. Except for a few written in Persian, all his works are in Arabic, which was considered as the language of science at the time. Thus it was a tradition for the scientists to write their in Arabic. Among his valuable books, the two most well-known books are *al-Shifa*, which deals mostly with philosophy, and the five-volume *al-Qānūn fi al-Tibb*, which is a complete medical encyclopedia.

Within less than a century, his book *Qānūn* was translated into Latin at the beginning of the 12th century and left a great impact on the Western medical world. This book was used as a course book in all European faculties of medicine, especially in Montpellier and Louvain Universities, which are the most famous medical faculties in France. Ibn Sina was the guide for medicine for Europe for 700 years. This went on until the middle of the 17th century. Ibn Sina not only influenced the Western world physicians but also philosophers and theologians with his work.

The significance of his books on medicine, especially the *Kanun (Qanun - Canon)*, in the Islamic world can be understood through the large number of the commentaries of the Arabic versions, and the translations and adaptations in Persian and Turkish. The influence of the *Qanun* in the West starts with the Latin translation done by Gerard from Cremona in Toledo. *Almagest* was also translated into Latin by Gerard in 1175.

It is understood that by the end of the 12th century, Greek Astronomy with the two sacred books of Greek-Arabic medicine assisted Latin scientists. From then on, almost all Latin medical books owe their knowledge of medicine to Ibn Sina. *Continens* and *Regalis Dispositio* were also printed by the first publishers; however, the success of these were not as much as that of *Qanun (Canon)*.

The well-known science historian George Sarton stated that, like Galen, who made a bibliography of his own works, Ibn Sina too did the same. Sarton adds that anybody writing as prolifically as they did would be lost towards the end of their lives without a comprehensive bibliography. In addition, Ibn Sina wrote *Qānūn al-Saghīr*, in the format of a short summary booklet, which gained fame after his death throughout the world and was used as a main course book and taught not only in medical schools in Europe and Anatolia, but also in the Islamic countries.

Life of Ibn Sina (980–1037)

Ibn Sina, by the time he was 20, had already studied the works of Aristotle, Euclid, Ptolemy (Batlamyus), and Galen, in addition to his religious education. During his youth in Buhara, he read lot of books written by al-Kindī (el-Kindi), Alpharabius (Al-Farabi), and Aristotle, which all were the source of his scientific curiosity. The works of Alpharabius (Al-Farabi), who was also known as "Magister Secundus" (Muallim-i Sani), explain the works of Aristotle. His passion for reading was inspired and encouraged by his father.

At the age of 18, Ibn Sina cured the Emir "Nuh II" of Buhara. Later on, he started to allocate more time for medicine. He was not only the Emir's physician but he was also his consultant. Ibn Sina lived for some time in Gorgan, Rey, Isfahan, and Hamadan. He cured another Emir, which caused the jealousy of his rivals, and as a result he had to endure torture. He was imprisoned for a while, yet fortunately he was allowed to write during his imprisonment. Later, he took shelter in Isfahan and spent the rest of his life there. Due to his assignment to accompany the army to Hamadan, he fell ill and died there in 1037 at the age of 57.

All his life he carried on his philosophical research alongside his scientific work. Clearly, Ibn Sina's contribution to humanity has been greater than his gains from the Indian, Greek, and Muslim worlds. His leadership in the field of philosophy and medicine continued for centuries. His significance lies not only in demonstrating solutions but also in how he approached problems. No other Muslim or Eastern scientist has ever had such a big impact on the world. Today, the portraits of the two Muslim physicians, Ibn Sina and Rhazes (Rāzī), hang in the Conference Hall of the Medical Faculty at Paris University near St. German Boulevard.

al-Qānūn fī al-Tibb

At the beginning of the 11th century, *al-Qānūn fī al-Tibb* was considered to be a synthesis of medical knowledge in experience and application, as it was established upon the bases formed by antique Greek scientists, like Hippocrates and Galen. It surpassed medical knowledge gained by the Byzantines and Arabs. Ibn Sina not only discovered the vast knowledge in Arabic works but he also knew how to benefit from the previous Arab syntheses. He also gathered most of the information in the works of Ebu Mansur Muwaffaq and the ones written by the Indian resources and incorporated them into his work. All this precious information was gathered and synthesized wisely and intelligently by him in his book *Qānūn*.

The word "Kanun" was derived from the Greek word 'canon' which means 'criteria'. The name was well-chosen because Ibn Sina's *Qānūn (Qanun)* was considered for six centuries as the medical criterion or a sacred book.

Qanun was divided into five main parts (volumes):

I. General topics (this part was mainly about medical philosophy)
II. Basic medicines in alphabetical order
III. Local diseases from head to toe
IV. General diseases like fever and others
V. Complex medicines (receipts)

Titles like Master of the Masters or other honorable titles given to him by Darü'l Islam (house of Islam) most probably were not given to him for his book *Shifa* (Cure) but for his book *Qanun*.

To understand the statements and concepts related to the causes of illnesses mentioned in the book, we need to know the main theory that guided all the physicians all over the world in humoral pathology, in that specific period of time the book was written. While reading the book, we come across the following terms: blood, bile, sputum, black bile or heat, coldness, moisture, and dryness or terms like "if it derived from the blood …fever from the bile which leads to headaches…pain which is caused by sputum and black bile…if pain is related to sputum, "sersam" illness caused by blood…, headache due to catching cold…".

Medieval medicine tries to explain that causes of illnesses are formed due to four main components and that the condition of illnesses depends on the amount of these components. Therefore, treatments focused on the improvement of the balance of these components. The "Theory of Humoral Pathology" considered these four main elements as the base, until Modern Medicine was widely accepted. Between 5th BC and 19th century AD, and by the second half of the 19th century when the "Cellular Theory", set forth by Rudolph Virchow, was widely accepted, this "Humoral Pathology Theory" received acceptance by all physicians for about 2500 years. According to Pythagoras (584–504 BC), the universe was formed by four main directions (North, South, East, and West); four main elements (fire, air, water, soil); four main physical features (heat, cold, dryness, and dampness); four products of nature (humans, animal, plant, and metal); and four seasons (spring, summer, autumn, and winter). Therefore, four has been the perfect symbol of inseparable interconnection with the earth.

Sicilian Empedocles (492–432 BC) is the first person to bring up the concept "Element" in his work called "Peri Physeos" (On the Nature). He formed the four-component theory that remained for about two thousand years. For

Empedocles, component means the matter that never changes by itself, in terms of quality, and is indivisible but can easily be transformed into various states.

The Universe (Cosmos)

Macrocosmos consists of these four components: earth, water, fire, and air. Being part of the universe (cosmos), humans (microcosmos) also contain the same components in certain proportions. These four components are unchangeable, indispensable, and immortal; when combined in different proportions, they cause various formations of beings in the universe. Therefore, all living and non-living things, which, of course, includes humans, are made up of these four main components. These also form flesh, blood, and other matters in humans and determine their "natura". This four-component theory of Empedocles would be used by the descendant scientists to explain the structure of beings in nature. The fact that this theory survived until the last century shows that change in scientific theories does not take place quickly. Another accepted main principle is "qualities". Everything existing in nature has "four main qualities", namely, heat, cold, dampness, and dryness. The four basic components forming nature also have the very same qualities. The components mentioned here should not be taken as fire, air, water, and soil in physical or chemical meaning. These are symbolic expressions of components/principles that are expressed in the same words in daily language: for example, cold or coldish which feels like cold. It should be considered as cold, heat, dryness, and dampness, which one feels in different seasons of the year.

This theory of Empedocles was accepted and applied to the human body by Hippocrates (460–377 BC). According to the so-called Humoral Pathology Theory, aliveness was made up of earth, forming the solid parts of the body; water, forming the liquid parts; air, enabling the respiration; and fire, which is the core of liveliness, i.e., the soul. There are four elements with different compositions, namely, liquid/humor: blood, sputum, yellow bile, and black bile. Each of these corresponding to air, water, earth, and fire has two properties: yellow bile corresponding to hot-dry fire; blood to hot-wet air; sputum to cold-wet water; black bile to cold-dry soil. Health depends on the equilibrium of the liquids in the body according to the person's nature. While some of these liquids, under certain circumstances, can change into another, some others do not.

For example, sputum can change into blood, blood can change into yellow bile, but blood does not change into sputum. As for black bile, it does not transform into any of these. Both the human body and the organs forming it come into being by mixing with these main elements in certain proportions.

The difference among them lies in the proportion of the mixtures. Therefore, each organ is different and carries different properties in its structure and hence has different characteristics. As an example, the heart and the liver are warm, the brain and bones are cold, the spinal cord and the lungs are humid, and hair has the quality of dryness. Considering these four elements and four qualities as the main principles without dispute, physicians did their medical practice for centuries. In humoral theory, “hilts” are the main elements of vital importance in the human body. These four main hilts (humor, liquid ore, liquid element, active liquid) are based on the thought that these four forms of liquid (blood, sputum, bile, and black bile) are present in blood. Health is the equilibrium of these four active liquid forms; diseases are the disorder of this balance. These four active liquids (blood, sputum, bile, and black bile) are formed like this: when food in the mouth is chewed, it is cooked and digested with heat and saliva; this is called the first digestion. The food moves to the stomach from the mouth; and with the heat and the substances, further digestion happens there. Here, the food takes a form like barley juice. This is called the second digestion (“keylus”; easily digested food). From here, some of the digested contents go to the bowels, the purest part is absorbed there, and the excess is removed from the bowels. Some goes to the liver. The digestion in the liver is the third digestion. All digested content gets treated in the liver, and the part which forms foam in blood and becomes bile. That, producing sediments in blood, becomes black bile. The undigested part in the blood is sputum, and the thoroughly digested part is blood. The center of blood is the heart and liver, the center of sputum is the brain, the center of bile is the liver, the center of black bile is the spleen and the stomach. These four basic liquid forms, which are of vital importance for the human body, have certain characteristics – blood: hot (warm) and damp; sputum: cold and damp; bile: hot and dry; black bile: cold and dry.

A human being is created with different proportional secretions of these four liquid substances. Even though these “hilts” show differences, they are gathered in four main groups. These are the ones with more blood “hilts”, sputum, black bile, or those with more bile hilts. This is called the nature (temperament). If blood humor is high, the person is called “sanguine” tempered. If sputum is high, he is “phlegmatic” tempered. If black bile is high, he is in “melancholy mood”. If bile is high, he is called to be a “bilious mood” type of human being.

Blood (hot/wet) is formed by good-quality food like meat and eggs, and in its overdose, there are symptoms such as bitterness in the mouth, sleepiness, stretching, yawning, itching where blood is drawn, slowing down in the actions of the body, pimples in the skin, nose bleeding, and skin rashes.

Bile (hot/dry) is formed by sugary food, and its excess causes a bitter taste in the mouth, thirst, paleness in the face, lack of appetite, and insomnia.

Sputum (cold/wet) is formed by fish, yoghurt, and raw fruit, and when it increases, indigestion, slowing down of the bodily actions, sleepiness, decline in body temperature are some possible outcomes.

Black bile (cold/dry) is formed by dry food like garlic; in excessive cases, lack of appetite, weight loss, pessimism, and complaints about nightmares occur.

A human being has a special nature according to the mixture of liquids in different percentages. Human nature tends towards one of these liquid matters. Therefore, in case we have more of one of the liquids in our body, our nature is also determined as warm-blooded (sanguine); calm, lazy/phlegmatic; outrageous, less lively/choleric; and pessimistic/melancholic.

Because seasons are the characteristics of the four basic elements, the food eaten in a season leads to diversity of the temperament. Summer is hot and dry – it increases the secretion of bile. Fall is cold and dry – it increases black bile. Winter is cold and wet – it increases the sputum. Spring is hot and wet – it increases blood. Physicians, on diagnosing a disease, practice their related treatment according to the patient's nature. The medicine for that illness has a different formula for those with sanguine, phlegmatic, melancholic, and choleric temperaments.

For this reason, it is very important for a physician to know the patient's nature. In addition, he needs to see blood, sputum, bile, and black bile as important; and he needs to know that the illness is caused by the disturbance of one of the humors, which the person has in a certain balance. He also needs to diagnose which humor has increased in that patient. Even though it is important for the physician to know the patient's temperament and which humors have been increased due to illness, he also needs to know another peculiarity, namely the property of that disease (i.e., hot, cold, damp, and dry). Every disease has one of the qualities of hot, cold, damp, and dry in a high amount.

On getting insight on the patient and the illness, the physician starts the treatment. The properties of the medicine resemble the humors causing the disease: hot, cold, dry, and damp. The treatment of the disease is to bring balance by increasing or reducing the disordered humors. This is possible with the medicine having reverse impact on the features of that humor. Therefore, it is essential to know all the qualities and features of each medicine. The properties of the medicine and food can be soothing, penetrating, anesthetic, or healing. It is necessary to know the above mentioned properties of the medicine and the diet and the substances to be used as medicine. For example, lettuce, lily, black night shade (*Solanum nigrum*), "mandrakes", opium are anesthetic; mallow (*Malva sylvestris*), marshmallow (*Althaea officinalis*), chard (*Beta vullgaris cicla*), "manna", and peanut are soothing; meat: strong and causing constipation; bean: laxative and water-absorbing; sea food: dry and light; cheese: strong and nutritious. Apart from this, saffron and laurel (*Louus nobilis*) are hot and dry, "sumac" is cold and dry, and apple is cold and damp.

According to Humoral Pathology theory, illnesses are believed to occur due to the imbalance in the arrangement of the four humors believed to exist in the body, for example, for a woman with delayed menstruation, to start menstruation, medicine soothing and relieving the stoppage is given; by giving the stone-removing medicine to the patient who is supposed to have a stone in the urethra; for psychological disorders by removing black bile or by improving it, the disordered balance will be brought to a healthy state.

Little Qanun (Kanun-u Sagir)

This is a ten-article book. By dividing it into subsections, in separate articles, first the creation of human being, the formation of the body and parts (fields) of medical sciences are explained in summary. The pulse is explained in detail. Urine, basic information about other organs of the body, the power of food and beverages; maintenance of health, education of children; guidance of pregnant and nursing women, illnesses of chest and abdomen and the part including both; stomach and the digestive system illnesses; urethral diseases; respiration arthralgia, malaria; accidental illnesses, bloodletting, poisonous insect stings are all explained in brief.

The following explanation of the expressions used in the book about food and medicine should be helpful for the readers.

The main properties of food and medicine are: light, dense, solid, fluid, sticky, dry, sweet, and fragrant.

The most frequently mentioned obvious impacts of food and medicine can be: relieving, comforting, solving, cutting (sharp), soothing, releasing, washing, solidifying, attractive, digestive, softening, blister-causing, gas repulsing, crushing, maturing, scraping, wound healing, stirring up, exterminating, strong, causing to rot, intensifying, padding, and causing to shrink, (defecating/removing), dissuasive, anesthetic, causing to be taut, strengthening, relieving, causing to fall, causing to remove stone, milk increasing, hindering milk secretion, brain-activating, etc.

I would like to state that we have had considerable difficulty in finding the corresponding lexis for certain vocabulary items while we, Dr. Ayhan Işık and Ekrem Sırma and I, Kadircan Keskinbora, were doing the translation, because the book was written in archaic Arabic 1000 years ago, and contained archaic Arabic terms and grammatical rules. We have also given the original names of the plants that we had difficulty to have access to translate. We have left a blank space for contradictory words and for those we have failed to clarify. Those we could not find the correspondents for are given in Arabic.

In this international symposium organized by Bahçeşehir University, we have decided to offer our participants a copy of the book mentioned above and registered in the catalogue Veliyüddin Efendi with the number 2529 in the "Hand Written Books" in the State Library, Bayezid, İstanbul, i.e., Ibn Sina's lesser known, handwritten book *El-Kitab El-Sagir*. Due to the support they have given for the decision to be put in practice, I would like to thank Prof. Dr. Türker Kılıç, the Dean of the Medical Faculty; our Rector Prof. Dr. Şenay Yalçın; and the Chairman of the Board of Trustees, Mr. Enver Yücel and Uğur Publishing for the efforts they have put forward in the meticulous design and visual quality of the book.

The book has been proofread several times. It has been also checked separately in terms of translation, editing, modification, simplification, and the relationship between subjects. I apologize to our readers for the errors we might have made in spite of all our painstaking efforts. Readers and scientists can send their comments, corrections, impressions, suggestions, and contributions, which I will appreciate to kadircan.keskinbora@gmail.com or hidirkadircan.keskinbora@med.bau.edu.tr

With the hope that the book will be a contribution to the Turkish medical, scientific, and cultural world,

Prof. Dr. Kadircan H. Keskinbora, M.D., Ph.D.

Second Edition Foreword (for Bahçeşehir Univ. edition)

It is obvious that lay people and scientists are in deep curiosity and express great interest towards Ibn Sina (Avicenna) and his books. This is evident by the fact that the first edition of Ibn Sina's *Little Qanun* was sold out in a year.

When we worked on the second edition, the first edition was looked through from the beginning to the end based on the notes I made on reviewing the first edition, according to the print and dictation errors, and feedback from readers. The statements are now more understandable in accordance to the main book's statements.

For a long time, English has been the international communicating language. So the translation in English will make it possible for the book to reach all the interested readers in the world. I have to thank Mrs. Serap Önsoy, who undertook the translation, for her disciplined and meticulous work. After the translation, we looked through the text word by word, sentence by sentence with regard to the medical terminology and medical English.

There may be some errors in this book, as may be in all books. I thank the readers in advance for their patience and generosity. For comments, contributions, and evaluations, the following e-mail addresses can be used:

hidirkadircan.keskinbora@med.bau.edu.tr or kadircan.keskinbora@gmail.com

Hoping that this book will contribute to science and humanity,

Prof. Dr. Kadircan H. Keskinbora, M.D., Ph.D.

Preface by the BAU Rector

The scientist, mathematician, philosopher, and physician whose full name being "Ebu Ali el-Hüseyin ibni Abdullah Ibn Sina el-Buharî" and shortly known as "İbn Sina" was born in Afshana near Buhara in today's Uzbekistan. He is known as "Avicenna" in Western sources and told to be as "Hâkim-i Tıb", i.e., master physician. All we know about him has been related by one of his loyal students "Ebu Ubeyd el-Cüzcani". He has recorded the life story told by "Ibn Sina" himself. Those who have told his life story have referred to this source.

As pointed out before "Ibn Sina" was born in Afshana, a village near Buhara, one of Horasan's big cities. His father was from the city of Belh and came to Buhara during the rule of Nuh ibn Mansur. He worked in local administration and became the ruler of the village Hermisan. His parents were married in Afshana near Hermisan. They settled there and his mother gave birth to Ibn Sina. Later they moved to Buhara.

During his lifetime, i.e., towards the end of the 10th century, in "Maveraunnehr" region "Samanoğulları (Samanids)" a Muslim state came to power during the decline and collapse of the state of Abbasi. Later in this geographical area, "Karahanlı (Karakhanids)" and "Gazneli (Ghaznevids)" Turkish States were founded. In short, this region was a cultural river basin where Turks met the Islamic religion and therefore Arabic, so Turkish and Persian cultures and customs interacted upon each other. Ibn Sina took his first education from his father and his older brother. Listening to their talks on the real self "nefs" and the mind, Ibn Sina first learns the Koran and literature and memorizes the Koran at the age of 10 and attends Ismail el-Zahid's law lectures. Ibn Sina understands these subjects deeply. Then he becomes the student of Ebu Abdullah el-Natili who is competent and an authority of philosophical topics and who comes to Buhara.

El Natili, being impressed by his explanations and intelligence, recommends Ibn Sina's father to lead him towards science. Learning the general subjects of the science of philosophy, Ibn Sina reads the philosophical books himself, and later becomes an expert in this field.

Ibn Sina who wants to learn the science of medicine reads the books related to the subject. He was, then, only 16 years old. Medicine is not a difficult science for him; in a short time he not only acquires the medical information, but he develops new methods of treatment and starts to cure his patients after receiving the title of physician at the age of 19. In a very short time, he surpasses his colleagues in this field. Treating and curing various patients, he achieves the wide spectrum of view about treatments not yet practiced. Alongside with medicine, he continues to study Islamic Law and its related issues and draws attention with his memory and diligence at a very young age. Meanwhile he also rescues Buhara Emir Nuh ibn Mansur from a severe illness, and therefore he receives permission to work in Samanogulları Palace Library. Thus, he achieves access to new studies and researches. Because of his expertise in philosophy, physics, and mathematics through his studies and success due to his superhuman efforts, he starts to be considered as "Şeyhu'r -Reis" (Master of the masters).

The period with the collapse of "Samanogulları (Samanids)" State and its division between "Karahanlılar (Karakhanids)" and "Gazneniler (Ghaznevids)" passes with historical fights in the form of struggle for dominance among Turkish and Muslim sovereigns. During this time, Ibn Sina rejects serving "Gazneli (Ghaznevids)" Emir Mahmud and lives in Urgenj, Merv, Nishabur, and Gurgan. A philosophy fan called Ebu Muhammed el Shiraz buys a house for Ibn Sina near his own in Gurgan, where he lives and writes his books with the names (El-Mebde' Ve'l-Mead) and 'El Ersadu'l - Külliye'. In addition to giving logic and astronomy lectures, he starts to write his book *al-Qānūn fi al-Tibb* during this term. Later he moves to Rey, Kazvin, and Hamadan, serving the local judges there. In that period of his life, he is brought to the post of vizierate for curing *Shams ad-Dawla* whose service he was in. However, he is sent to prison in a rebel against him. The Emir sends him to exile. During this time, he starts to write his well-known work *el-Shifa*. Later, going to Isfahan Ibn Sina goes under the service of Emir *Ala ad-Dawla*.

The Emir flatters him a lot and he completes writing *el-Shifa*. Then he writes *En-Necat*. He goes to Hamadan where he writes *Danishname-i Alai* in Persian. His work "Lisan'ul Arab" remains incomplete in a draft form. His student "Cüzcani" states that Ibn Sina was strong in every subject. When he suffers from severe pains in his shoulder, he treats him in a quick and intensive way. Even though he applies treatments eight times a day, Ibn Sina's body falls weak. When the illness spreads throughout his body, he stops the treatment. After a few days, at the age of 57 in (1037 June–July) he dies in Hamadan where his grave is situated.

The information about Ibn Sina's works differs. Ibn Hallikan, Kıfti, Useybiya, and other sources give different information on the number of his works. As for "Kâtip Çelebi", he rerecords his 57 works in different volumes. One of the two studies on this matter is that of Yahya Mehdavî's Fihrist (Tehran, 1954) and the other is the one which is based on Ibn Sina's works in Turkey with the name 'Müellefatu Ibn Sina el Mahtutat fi Turkey' (Cairo, 1973). These two sources are considered reliable. The names of 131 works, which definitely belong to Ibn Sina, are listed in "Hayrani Altıntash's" book. "Mehdavî" adds 111 works more to these works. Anawati, however, gives the name of 276 works. As for Ibn Sina's work *al-Qānūn fi al-Tibb* (The law of medicine is known shortly as "Kanun") – this book including the medical knowledge of its time was used as a course book for 400 years in the West and was considered to have overtaken the reputation of early Greek authorities: Hippocrates and Galen.

The Picture of the cover of the Latin publication of *al-Qānūn fi al-Tibb* (Pavia, 1510) is an illustration (depiction) of how his authority in medicine is evaluated; because the Picture depicts Ibn Sina on a throne in the middle and Hippocrates and Galen sitting on either side of him. Ten Latin translations of *Qanun* have been done; the work has been divided into different branches such as physiology, hygiene, therapeutics, and pharmacology. While he was doing researches in medicine, he sensed that some invisible creatures played a role in passing down some illnesses to a human, i.e., he sensed the existence of microbes (microbiological entities), and he often mentioned these unknown creatures in his works. When *al-Qānūn fi al-Tibb* was translated into Latin in the 12th century, it had a great impact on the Western medical world and became the main course book of the most famous medical schools of Montpellier and Louvain Universities.

This situation continued until the middle of the 17th century. An Ibn Sina (Avicenna) desk was founded in Valladolid University. Ibn Sina was the medical professor of Europe for 700 years. He wrote some of his books in Persian, most being in Arabic. The place in which Ibn Sina lived was Turkish lands; however, in the reign of "Karahanlılar (Karakhanids)", it is seen that Turkish was vastly used, and classical works of Turkish language were produced. However, Persian and Arabic started to become the language of Turkish states along with "Gazneliler (Ghaznevids)". Turkish scientists wrote their works in these languages. During the following "Selçuklular (Seljuqs)" reign, Turkish history slides to Iranian geography and therefore Persian became the language of administration. Therefore, Ibn Sina, who is known as a Persian physician and philosopher, also has poems which he wrote in Turkish. Moreover, Ibn Sina also leaves his trace in Turkish folk stories. Stories from Ibn Sina were collected in a book and presented to Ottoman Emperor Murad the third (his reign between 1574 and 1595) by a person named "Dervish Hasan Mahdi". The various issues of these stories are observed in Anatolian Turkish folk culture (folklore). These were introduced by Ahmet Ateş, Saim Sakaoğlu, Mehmet Çayırdağ, and Doğan Kaya. On the other hand, in Iranian and Latin literature around his name long stories and legends are seen to be told. We owe our deepest thanks to the Symposium Organization Committee for enabling us, within the premises of Bahçeşehir University, to commemorate the great scientist Ibn Sina, who is and will always be mentioned about his great contributions to the world of medicine. Our many thanks also goes to our teacher, Prof. Dr. Kadircan Keskinbora, who has realized the translation of this souvenir book and who has made it possible for the book to be introduced to the scientific and cultural world, and we acknowledge the assistance of our BAU Medical School Dean, Prof. Dr. Türker KILIÇ.

Prof. Dr. Şenay Yalçın
Rector, BAU

Preface by the Dean of the BAU School of Medicine

Ibn Sina, with his medical profession, rationalism, and experimentalism and along with his not only scientific but also metaphysical interpretation, has contributed unforgettable pages to the history of medicine and philosophy. It is obvious how much impact he and others like him have had on the world culture. Even though one thousand years have passed since his birth, Ibn Sina still survives. On related matters, he is always mentioned in books and conferences in different parts of the world. We, Bahçeşehir University and the Medical School, feel the great honor of the fact that our symposium is held as the celebration of the 1000th anniversary of the completion of *Kanun* and as a sign of the importance given to Ibn Sina, who has had an important place in our culture for 1000 years, and of the translation and presentation of this book to the medical world. I would like to thank our scientific and social committees who have organized and realized the symposium, and our university teaching staff member, Dr. Kadircan Keskinbora, who has enabled this work to be translated and presented to the world of science and culture.

Prof. Dr.Türker Kılıç
Dean, Bahçeşehir University Medical School

Contents

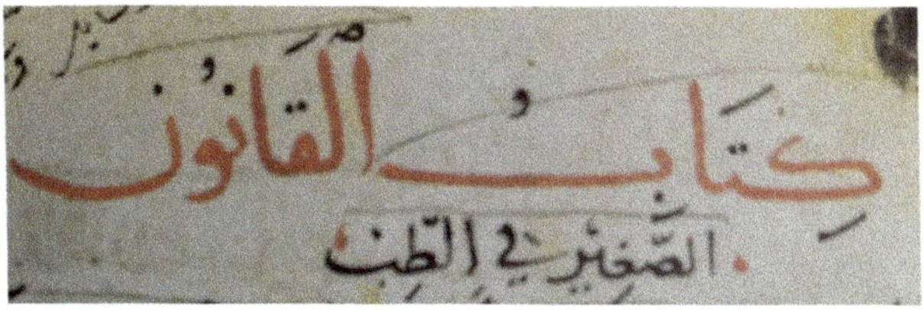

God bless him

Mustensikh:

The person who transcribed and copied the book is Ibn Huruf was born in Salti, live in Tripoli and known as Sheikh Abdul Wahab Bin Ibrahim, may God bless his soul, the people who pray for him and all Moslems.

Introduction[1]

In the name of Allah, Most Gracious, Most Merciful. God, help me finish this book in good faith. Praise be to the most wonderful words said by God, and His blessing be on His subject and prophet Muhammad in the purest and most gracious way.

The interest for science is bestowed (given) by Mighty God to those of maturity and integrity; and to those with pure hearts, clear eyes, and the self-confidence to carry on the work.

Mighty God has chosen you as the best and most mature man to be endowed with wide scientific knowledge. As a man who values science, and a benevolent teacher, may you get in return even more than you have given to your students in knowledge and affection.

Upon Your instructions, my publications on medicine will be written in clear expressions, concise explanations, and language that would be easily understood by everyone, at all times. They will provide benefits for all conditions and ailments. With God's help I will fulfill the mission that has been entrusted to me. Success is God's will.

This book consists of ten articles.

---

1 Kanun-u Sagir looks like a little model, not a summary of *al-Kanun fi't-Tibb*. This introduction has been organized similar to his introduction of his main book (*Great Qanun*) where Ibn Sina addresses himself.

[2A] (Contents)[2]

The first article

This article is about the creation of the human being, the structure of the body, the sections (components) of the science of medicine, the pulse, urine, and information about the other organs. There are seven chapters:

1. The creation of the human being
2. The structure of the human body from separate organs (parts)
3. The structure of the body from compound pieces (organs in groups)
4. The different sections of the science of medicine – their descriptions and importance
5. The flow of blood through the vessels
6. The urine
7. Information about the other parts of the body

The second article

This article is about the function and energy of food, beverages (drinks), and clothes (fabrics). There are twenty chapters:

1. Bread and bread types
2. Meat and eggs
3. Fish
4. Milk, cream, fat, butter, and cheese
5. Legumes
6. Other legumes
7. Fresh fruit
8. Dry food
9. Fats (oils)
10. Aromatic plants (herbs) (Reyahin)
11. Fragrances
12. Clothes (fabrics)
13. Spices
14. Vinegar, olive, baudha (boza, beverage made of fermented millet), pickles, and jams

---

2 Ibn Sina's original book does not have the contents in his book, but he wrote the titles and the summaries of his article at the beginning. This content list is arranged by myself.

15. Oral acnes
16. How to brighten the teeth and make the mouth smell nice (avoid bad breath)
17. Uvula (epiglottis), the swelling of tonsils in the throat
18. Secretions of mucus (phlegm/sputum) in the throat

The fifth article

Illnesses related to the chest down to the abdomen. There are four chapters:

1. Coughs, colds, and pleurisy
2. Asthma
3. Palpitations
4. Blood in the saliva (hemoptysis)

The sixth article

This article is about abdominal illnesses and their relations to food and nutrition.

There are fourteen chapters:

1. Stomach weaknesses (diseases)
2. Nausea
3. Colic
4. Hiccups
5. Diarrhea
6. Dysentery
7. Gripes
8. Abdominal worms
9. Liver pains
10. Spleen pains
11. Jaundice
12. Kidney diseases
13. Bladder diseases
14. Anus diseases

The seventh article

This article is about the diseases of the genital organs. There are six chapters:

1. Penis (male organ) diseases
2. The discharge of seminal fluid and semen
3. Testicle (testis) diseases
4. Hernia
5. Womb (uterus) diseases
6. Sexual intercourse

[4A] The first article

Chapter one: Regarding the creation of the human being

The aim of the study of science is to keep the human body healthy the way it was created. When an illness occurs, science should be able to cure the body from that specific illness and return it to its healthy state. For that reason, a physician should know the human body well, and he should also know each and every single detail related to the changes that have taken place because of the illness, so as to be able to bring the body back to its healthy state.

So we can refer to the Greek physicians' claim that, when a healthy and strong flow of water (semen) and sperms reach the womb of the woman and settles there firmly, the womb has the chance to be inseminated/fertilized; and, at the same time, if the woman's womb is healthy and without any illness, then, according to our belief and with the will of Mighty God, the insemination will take place and the woman will become pregnant.

According to the Greek doctors, a baby is created from the combination of the man and woman's liquids. However, if the two liquids or one of them is damaged or weak, no baby can develop. In addition, if there is a problem in the womb, or after intercourse, even if the liquids and the womb of the woman are both healthy, a harsh and uncomfortable movement from the man towards the woman's womb at that moment can cause the liquids to slip away, so pregnancy will not take place.

Some physicians claim that, during the first two weeks after insemination, the liquids become a blood clot (alaq), and in three weeks that becomes a morsel of flesh (mudgha). With this, the creation of a human being will take place. The creation of a male takes 30–40 days, whereas, the creation of a female takes 40–50 days. During the creation period, the fetus doubles its constant movements/activity, and the baby will be born at the end of the period when it triples the days of its movements/activity. If the creation of a fetus is completed in 35 days, then it will be active for 70 days and will be born at the end of 210 days. The baby will be in the group of children who are born in their seventh month. If the creation of the fetus is completed in 40 days, then it will move for 80 days and will be born at the end of 240 days. The baby will be in the group of children who are born in their eighth month; in which case, it is assumed that the fetus cannot survive. For the ones whose creation takes 45 days and constant movements 90 days, birth will take place in 270 days. These babies are considered to be in the group that will be born in nine months.

The reason given for why a seven-month-old baby can survive after birth, but an eight month-old baby cannot, is based on Hippocrates' explanations. In his book about the newborn child, he says when a fetus that has completed its sixth month and is in its seventh month and makes a harsh movement, it can abort from its natural passage against its will. If the fetus is healthy, strong, and robust, it can overcome all the obstacles and get to the other side of the womb and be born. In this kind of birth, the baby can survive. Even though an eight-month-old baby is more perfect and lasting than a seven-month-old, if he/she is thin, weak, and not strong enough, he/she will be ill and will keep being unhealthy and ill in the womb in his/her eighth month. If this illness is not serious, he/she will complete the eighth month and enter the ninth month, which means that he/she can survive. But if the illness is severe he/she will die. His/her death will either take place in the womb and be stillborn, or he/she could be born ill, and die afterwards because the changes in the environment will increase his/her illness which will lead to his/her death.

Chapter two: The organs that build up the human body

The human body is made of single and compound organs (systems). With the help of God, we will talk about the compound organs (systems) after finishing our talk about individual organs.

Individual organs

They are bones, nerves, ligaments (ribataat), tendons (ewtaar), muscles, vessels, arteries, veins, fat, membrane, skin, hair, and finger nails.

Bones

One of the bones is the skull, and it is composed of seven skull bones which are called "qabayil el re's". Some of the bones are the subdivisions of the other parts and they are called the "shun".

- The upper jaw is composed of 18 bones.
- The lower jaw is composed of two bones.
- The rest are the teeth. There are 32 teeth, 16 on each jaw: the incisors, the drillers, (canines and premolars), and molar teeth. Each half jaw has five molar teeth.
- The neck vertebra is composed of seven bones.

- The thorax (chest) is composed of 17 vertebras. It is also called the ribcage. There are 24 ribs.
- The back (dorsum) is made of seven vertebras.
- The collarbone is composed of two bones.
- Each shoulder is composed of two bones.
- Each arm is composed of a humerus, an ulna, and eight more bones, and the wrist.
- The hand consists of four bones.
- Five fingers consist of 15 bones.
- The hips consist of two bones.
- Each thigh has two bones, and each leg has two bones, too.
- Each foot is made of a heel, an arch, and a bone which is called the caique (boat bone). The ankle has four bones, and there are four bones at the ball of the foot. The five toes have 28 bones.
- The total bones in the human body is 248.

These bones have two benefits for the body: the first is to keep the body in the erect position, and the second is to protect and provide the body's continuity.

Similarly, as Mighty God's creation, the hipbone, the coccyx bone, and the spine are made to fundamentally support the other organs. For some others, these bones are the shields that protect the organs. This is clearly seen in the case of how the skull protects the brain and how the rib cage protects the heart. The same situation can be considered in the relationship of the ribs and the lungs, as the ribs' function is to protect the lungs.

The nerves (the nervous system)

The function of nerves in the body is to make the body feel and accordingly be able to move. These movements and senses are of two types:

The first type is derived from the brain (dimagh). This is in seven pairs, which give the five senses and the other organs' sense and movement.

The second type is derived from the bottom part of the brain (nukha'). This part has 31 pairs, but one of these is single and it does not have a pair. These types of nerves with their organ connections up to the neck form the senses and their movements.

The muscles

The muscles are the flesh of the body. They consist of only flesh, nerves, and vessels. They help the body in two ways. First, with the help of the tendons, they allow the joints to move and cover all bones like a garment. The other benefit is to prevent the body from getting cold by protecting the natural temperature of the body.

The arteries

The arteries are linked to the heart. They consist of nerves with multilayers. Basically, they are without sense or movement. With lots of energy and very little blood. Yet the arteries' benefit is to give the organs the power of life.

The veins

The source of the veins is the liver. They do not have multilayers. Basically, they are without sense or movement. They are streams of the liver. They have a lot of blood but very little energy. Their function is to carry blood from the liver to the organs.

The fat

The fat is the lipid in the thorax and in the intestine. Its function is to provide body temperature and to increase the power of protection in the body. Another fat is the kidney fat. Its function is to protect the two kidneys from diseases.

The sensory organs

The sensory organs are neural bodies. They are hard, thin, and have no sense or movement. Their function is to protect the organs.

The skin

The skin, similar to the brain (the dimagh), is a neural body. Its function is to cover the flesh and protect it. The skin has also a lot of stomas (pores). These pores are the places where hair is found and where sweat and pleasant vapors can exit from. In this way, the body breathes.

Hair

There are four kinds of hair: the kind which makes the body attractive (decorates the body) and is a protective cover at the same time. Head hair is one example because it protects the head skin and also decorates the whole body.

Some hair only decorates the body and some only provides benefits to some organs, such as the eyebrows and the eyelashes. These can protect the eyes from diseases and also can increase their strength. They add beauty to the whole body. Some hair kinds provide only benefits and do not have any decorative functions. These kinds are on the rest of the body; their function is to get rid of body waste.

The nails

The nails are neural and have hard plates without sense. Nails have two functions: the first is to cover the upper edge of the fingers and support the fingers to hold and use objects. Also they help the flesh on the upper part of the fingers by supporting and strengthening them. When the fingers hold objects, the nails support them and provide the necessary help to hold them. The second function is to use the nails as a weapon by human beings and other animals. In addition, they also fulfill the function of a knife for human beings.

Chapter three: It is about the structure of the body from compound systems

The compound organs (systems) are: the brain (dimagh), the two eyes, the tongue, the ears, the heart, the lungs, the eyebrows, the eyelashes, the breast, the thorax, the abdomen, the stomach, the intestines, the liver, the bile, the spleen, the kidneys, the urinary tract, the testes, the penis, the uterus (womb), and the joints.

The brain

The essence of the brain (dimagh) is cerebral, yet it is harder and less fatty than the outer brain cortex. It is a white, thin, loose, and shaky substance. The brain (dimagh) being cerebral contains veins, vessels, and arteries, and also has a fine marrow-like membrane called the "protector of the brain" (simhak). Just at the back of the dimagh and the skull is the place where the cerebellum and medulla spinalis are located. It is exactly like the dimagh in the shape of a triangle but not exactly in a triangular shape.

The basis of this triangle is the line that connects the front part of the head with the shinbone at the back (rear) part of the head. The senses are carried through the soft nerves, and activities are carried through the hard nerves. The brain has cavities which contain the psychoactive spirit. Thinking, perception of life, shapes, and visualization of objects takes place at the front part of the brain. The rear part of the brain is the place where memorization and understanding takes place. According to Hippocrates, the brain is the first organ in the human body.

The eyes

Each eye has seven layers and three types of liquids. The first layer is associated to the air. It is called the conjunctiva (Al tabaqa el-multahime). This is the white part of the eye. The second layer is the cornea (Al tabaqa al-Qarniyye). The color of the cornea differs from one person to the other. Sometimes it is black, blue, or hazel. Then comes the vitreous fluid (Al rutuba al-baydhiye). This fluid is similar to egg white. After that, there is the arachnoid layer (Al tabaqa al-ankebutiye). This layer resembles the spider web texture in its softness. The following layer is the lens – glacier moisture layer (Al rutuba al-jelidiyye). This fluid is pure bright. It looks like an ice layer but with incomplete roundness. After that comes the vitreous fluid, the glassy fluid (Al rutuba al-zujaciyye) which functions like a glass window in connection to sight. The next layer is the retina (Al tabaqa al-shebekiyye). This layer looks like a knitting pattern. The following layer is the choroidea layer (Al tabaqa al-meshimiyye); it is similar to the placenta, as both of them have lots of vessels. The last layer is a hard layer on the eye bone, the sclera (Al tabaqa al-sulbe). The eyes rest on their sockets.

The tongue

The tongue consists of thin white flesh, veins and arteries, and a major nerve. It is very sensitive. In fact, it consists of consecutive muscles and skin, which adjoins the esophagus and the stomach skin. The main functions of the tongue are: speaking, chewing food, and assisting in swallowing.

The ears

The ears consist of cartilage, pure flesh, and sensitive nerves. Hearing functions through the auditory canal (al sama'). The ear receives the sounds, and slowly allows them to enter the auditory canal.

The heart

The heart is in the shape of a cone. It is located in the middle of the chest cavity, with a base leaning to the left, in eye-catching red color. The inner part of the heart is a combination of fiber-like substance and a hard membrane called the El shugaf. The heart has two chambers: the right one has a lot of blood but little energy, and the left one has a lot of energy but little blood. There is a transition for the flow from both parts to one another. From these the veins and arteries appear. At the right side of the heart, the flow channels are found. Through these channels, the nutrient blood flows from the heart to the lungs and, accordingly, inhalation will flow from the lungs to the heart. The heart is the source of natural heat (caloric) energy and animal spirit. According to Aristotle and Galen, the heart is the first organ that is created in the human body.

The lungs

The lungs are rose-colored, thin pieces of flesh. The flow of blood starts from the tube to the two lungs and from there through the tissues throughout the lungs. Vessels, which are not arteries, carry blood and energy from the heart. It is impossible to find any kinds of senses in the lungs. They are covered with very fine membrane. The lungs have tubes and minor tubules. The function of the lungs is to maintain the natural heat in the heart and to protect the heart by surrounding it.

The thorax

The thoracic diaphragm (hijab) is a neural substance. Though this compound consists of flesh in its origin, there is no flesh in the middle part. Sensitive and active nerves that are bigger than the "dimagh" make up the diaphragm, which collects blood and makes the heartbeat.

The stomach

The stomach which has a circular shape consists of nerves, flesh, vessels, and arteries. The fleshy side is in its cavity and its neck. There is no flesh at the outlet of the stomach. The stomach has three parts: the esophagus, the gastric outlet, and the stomach cavity. The esophagus starts at the end point of the mouth and ends at the breastbone, which is attached to the end part of the chest tube.

The outlet of the stomach is located at the intersection of the thorax and shows immediate response when touched under the soft bone. The real location of the stomach cavity is above the umbilicus slightly inclined to the left.

The intestines

There are six intestines. Three are thin and three are thick. They are located near the left side of the involvement of pleurisy and the stomach. They are also shaky and look like the liver. Their color is matt. The inside part is hollow and the membrane has sensitive neural layers. Their function is to eliminate (expel) food (intestinal) waste.

The spleen

The spleen is located between the ribs and the left part of the stomach, with a loose (flabby) structure. Both the spleen and the liver have the same flesh. It has a matt color with no sense but its webs are highly sentient. (The spleen is the storage of black bile. Its function is to draw the black bile out of the liver.)

The liver

The location of the liver is on the right side of the body. The upper part of the liver is webbed by pleura. The back (rear) side of it is attached to the ribs. The ventral side is attached to the rear (back) ribs and the stomach, and the bottom side is attached to the thigh (hip). The color of the liver is dark red and looks like clotted blood.

The liver is the starting point of the veins and the main source of energy (strength). It consists of membrane, artery, vein, and canals. There is no sense in its essence, whereas, there is great energy (strength) in the webs. Its function is to produce blood for the body.

The bile

The bile is attached to the liver. It is the pot for the yellow poison. Its function is to draw the yellow poison out of the liver.

The kidneys

The kidneys are located at the bottom part of the dorsal leaning on the spine. Each one of them is solid, reddish, and has fatty flesh, veins, and arteries, with no sense but its webs are highly sentient. Their function is to draw the urine out of the liver whose vessels send the urine to the bladder.

The bladder

The bladder is located between the anus and the lower abdomen. Its body is covered with spotless flesh and consists of neural layers, veins, and arteries. Its function is to store the urine and stop it from being involuntarily discharged.

The testes

The main substance of the testes is white fat. They look like fatty flesh but smaller, softer, and whiter and consist of veins and arteries which are all covered by a web.

Their function is to mature the semen and prepare them to be used when the time comes.

The penis

The penis consists of lots of nerves, veins, arteries, and layers of muscles. It has a strong sense of feeling. Its function is well known.

The uterus (womb)

The uterus (womb) is also a neural body. It is located between the bladder and the rectum. The cervix is long and ends at the sexual organ. On the two sides of the womb, there are two eggs at the base of its horns. It is neural and very sensitive and consists of veins and arteries. Its function is to accept pregnancy.

The joints

The joints are found in the head, the neck, the two shoulders, the two collars, the hip, the thigh, the legs, and the feet. The four elements of the body are mentioned and discussed in Chapter nine.

Chapter four: The sections of medical science and their explanations

Medical science is divided into two branches: theoretical and practical.

The theoretical branch is the fundamental one, which is the science and knowledge of the natural and the nonnatural.

The data of the external and nonfundamental things:

There are 11 elements that form the basics:

I) Fire, air, water, and earth
   Fire is hot and dry. Air is hot and wet. Water is cold and wet. Earth is cold and dry.
II) Secretions and excretions (four kinds)
   1. Blood that is hot and wet
   2. Yellow bile that is hot and dry
   3. Black bile that is cold and dry
   4. The sputum that is cold and wet
III) The third one is divided into nine. The first four are:
   1. Heat
   2. Coldness
   3. Wetness
   4. Dryness

   The other four are:

a. Heat-dryness
b. Heat-wetness
c. Coldness-dryness
d. Coldness-wetness
e. The ninth combination is the one in the middle, which is the moderate.

IV) The fourth is the organs that we have covered under Chapters two and three.

V) The fifth is the organs' potential energy. Each one has its own potential energy. For example, flesh is hot and wet, bones are cold and dry, and nerves are cold and wet.
The compound organs also have their own potential energy. For example, the brain (dimagh) is cold and wet. The heart is hot and wet. The liver is hot and wet. The bile is hot and dry. The spleen is cold and dry.
Every organ has its innate potential energy. One of these is attraction; this energy attracts the necessary nutrition towards the organ. The second is getting hold of (upholding) potential energy in which the organ holds and protects whatever it has attracted. The third one is digestion and assimilation – these digest the food. The fourth is the defensive potential energy which protects the organs from excessive food and other things.

VI) The sixth is the functions of the organs' functions. For example, the bile attracts the food. The stomach digests the food. The intestine provides the transportation of the food.

VII) The seventh is the essences. One of them is the psychological essence, which is located in the brain (dimagh). The other is the animal essence, which is located in the heart.

VIII) The eighth is the human being himself, divided into four stages:
1. Childhood is hot and wet.
2. Youth is hot and dry.
3. Maturity is cold and dry.
4. Old age is cold and wet from the age point of view, and cold and dry from the organs' point of view.

IX) The ninth is the colors. Sputum is white, blood is red, yellow bile is yellow, and black bile is black.

X) The tenth is fat. This is when the body is overweight or underweight. If the excess weight is from the fat, then it is hot and wet. If it is only the flesh, then it is hot and wet, and if it includes the paleness then it is cold and dry.

XI) The eleventh is the differences between the male and female. The male, in general, is hot; and the female, in general, is cold.

The innate ones are nine:

1. The air that surrounds the body
2. The temperature
3. Tranquility/peace
4. Taking a bath
5. Food
6. Drinks/beverages
7. Sleep
8. Being awake
9. Personal moods and reactions: happiness, sadness, anger, and satisfaction

There are three unnatural states or conditions:

1) Sicknesses
2) Knowing (learning) the reasons for these sicknesses
3) Knowing their symptoms

The function of medical science has two divisions:

A) It protects healthy people from illnesses
B) It cures them from diseases

Medical science is defined as:

1) Knowing matters that prevent diseases and provide health
2) Knowing matters that protect from diseases or what causes these diseases
3) Studying situations that are not related to health or illnesses

There are three different types of masters involved in medical science:

1) The ones who know and can interpret and compare with experience
2) The ones who do not have any notion and cannot compare without experience
3) A group of people who use tricks and are fraud

Chapter five: Brief information related to the pulsing of the vessels

All the vessels proportionally follow the heartbeat. For that reason, it is possible to get the heartbeat from any vessels in the body.

The best locations to obtain the pulse are the wrists, the temples, and the ankles where the arteries are most visible. Whereas, inside the body, the best place to get the beat of the pulse is from the vessels that are located under the left heart cavity, as this is the first artery that leaves the heart. The beats of the arteries that are found inside the spine can only be felt by touching the belly.[3]

There are ten types of pulses and those ten types have their own varieties:

I) The first kind is related to the expansion and the contraction of the vessels: the long pulse, the wide pulse, and the moderate pulse.
   a. The long pulse beats (its movement) can be felt under the fingers, and it can be felt on a wider surface of the finger. It indicates high fever. This is found in slim bodies.
   b. The wide pulse, which takes place in the wide part of the fingers, is bigger than the moderate pulse. This indicates high humidity.
   c. The moderate pulse is the one which is between the others, and it indicates that the heat and coldness, the humidity and the dryness in the body is stable.

II) The second kind of pulse/heartbeat is related to the ways of movement. These are also of three types. One of them is rapid, the other is slow, and the last one in between is the moderate one.
   a. The rapid pulse is the one that hits the fingertips excessively. This indicates that the heart is in need of cold air.
   b. The slow pulse is the one that hits the fingertips slowly. This indicates that the heart is in low temperature.
   c. The moderate pulse indicates the stable heart condition.

III) The third kind is related to the force of the pulse. This is also of three types: strong, weak, and moderate.
   a. The strong pulse is the one that hits the fingertips hard, up to its depth. This indicates animal-like strength.
   b. The weak pulse, on the other hand, indicates the weak condition of animal-like strength.
   c. The moderate pulse is the one in between which indicates the moderate condition of animal-like strength.

IV) The fourth kind is related to the density (physical structure) of the arteries. This is also of three types. One is hard, the other is soft, and the third one, in between, is moderate.
   a. The hard type is the one when the vessel is touched by the fingertips is hardly affected. This indicates that the body is dry.
   b. The soft type is the one when the vessel is touched by the fingertips is strongly affected. This indicates that the body is soft and has a lot of moisture.

---

3 He means abdominal aorta.

c. The moderate type is the one in between and indicates that the body is stable in dryness and softness.

V) The fifth kind is related to fatigue in the movement. This is also of three types:

a. The continuous pulse that is felt on the fingertips nonstop indicates weakening in strength. The pulse gets bigger when it is continuous, but when there are occasional interruptions, it indicates that there is something unusual in the body.
b. The second one is the one with mixed beats. This type is sluggish (with slow rhythm), which indicates that the body is cold. Sometimes when it is irregular or low, it indicates weakness in strength.
c. The third one is the moderate one that is between the other two, as we explained before.

VI) The sixth kind is related to the order of the pulse. This type arranges and protects the beat to be in one order. This indicates that the body is in good condition.

VII) The seventh kind is related to the varieties/irregularities. This is when the pulse varies and is changeable, indicating that the body is in an unstable condition.

VIII) The eighth kind is related to the slowness of the movement. In this type of beat, the pulse should be parallel with the calmness of the body. This indicates that the body is stable during the expansion and the tightening of the vessels.

IX) The ninth kind is related to the types of heat and the coldness of the arteries. They are of three types.

a. The first one is being hot. The vessel, itself, should also be hot. This indicates the temperature of blood and energy in the vessel.
b. The second one is being cold. This means that the arteries have to be cold. This indicates lack of blood and energy in the vessel.
c. The third is the moderate one. This indicates the stability in the condition of the energy in the heat and the coldness.

X) The tenth kind is related to the contents within the arteries. They are also of three types.[4]

a. The full ones indicate that there is a lot of blood and energy in them.
b. The hollow ones indicate that blood and energy in the vessels are in stable condition.

4 There is no third type in the original copy.

Chapter six: Brief and basic information related to urine and urethra

Urine could indicate one of two things: Either common illnesses like the malaria, which irritate the body, or other illnesses in the urethra that covers the kidneys, through the penis for the male and through the vagina for the females.

The stable urine is the urine in good condition.

The urine is divided into two parts:

1) Water
2) The sediment that is thicker than the water

Water is of two types:

a. The degree of density
b. The color
c. The degree of density is of three types: the first one is delicate (thin), the other is dense, and the third one is moderate.
d. The color is of six types:
    1. The first one is white.
    2. The second one is yellow, which is the color of citrus.
    3. The third one is the color of the fire, and it is more yellowish than orange.
    4. The fourth is light red, which is the color of "Zaferaan" (saffron) hair.
    5. The fifth is dark red, which is the color of blood.
    6. The sixth is the black color.

The white urine is the result of either indigestion or due to too much sputum in the urine.

When the urine contains some bile, the color will change into orange. The light red color is due to the urine containing too much bile.

The dark red color is due to the urine containing blood.

The black color urine sometimes is caused by extreme coldness, which destroys the heat, and sometimes it is caused by the extreme heat, and some other time it is caused by black bile mixed in the urine.

The urine that contains a mixture of white and yellow is the moderate one. Inside the urine, there is white mass sediment.

1) There are four types of urine sediment analysis:
    a. The first is the color.
    b. The second is the position (place).
    c. The third is the consistency (density).
    d. The fourth is the timing of when it is seen.

a. The color: any color apart from white indicates that there is some kind of disorder in the body.
b. When it comes to its position, only the urine at the bottom of the flask is bad.
c. When it comes to density, if the urine is either too high or too low, then this is also bad.
d. The time the urine is passed is always important in healthy bodies. Disorders appear in the urine of patients, either at the beginning of the illness or after some time. When the urine is passed, it means that the patient is recovering and the illness is rapidly fading away, but when the urine is not easily passed, then, it means that the illness is not in its recovery period.

Chapter seven: Conditions of secretions and excretions of the body (elimination of waste)

With the will of God to keep the body healthy, it is necessary to throw away the waste from the body every day.

1) The first waste that the body should eliminate is the food waste. It is important to do this every day to keep the body healthy. The stomach, the whole intestine, and the hollow parts of the liver can be healthy only when the discharging takes place. This excretion should take place at the same hour every day. The excrement should be between soft and hard (semisolid). Also, as it was discussed before in the topic of moderate urine, and moderate bile, it should be light yellow in color with not much odor.
2) The second is the urine. It is necessary to discharge the urine completely. This action is necessary for the safety of the dry part of the liver, the kidneys, the bladder, and the whole urinary tract.
3) The third is sweat. Sweat is a kind of urine. The proof is its color, as the color of urine is yellow and it smells bad. This should be discharged every day. This action is necessary for the safety of the vessels and beyond the vessels, the flesh and the skin.
4) The fourth is the other organs. The brain discharges its waste from the nostrils as mucus and from the mouth as sputum. The waste from the chest and the lungs is discharged through breathing.

Apart from that, there are other wastes that are discharged by passing air or by discharging waste (defecating) through the anus. These are three kinds: noisy, rapid, and silent.

Discharging waste (defecating) with noise shows that the intestine has discharged all the feces (waste), and that there is nothing left behind except air. And discharging with loud noise shows that the waste from the intestines is a mixture of sputum, humidity, and rough air.

If the silently discharged waste is difficult to be discharged, this means that the residue is coming down. Yet if the odor is distinctive, this shows that there is some digestion problem. Also it shows that the food residue has bad smell. For example, when garlic, onion, leeks, and all the types of beans with bad smell are eaten either fried or uncooked, their residue would smell very bad. It is easier to discharge waste with no odor. This would show healthy digestion and a clean stomach.

The end of the first article.

[17A] The second article

This chapter is related to the energy of food and beverages.[5]

Chapter one: The energy of the grains

Wheat is first-degree hot, wet, and highly nutritional.

Barley is first-degree cold and dry, low in nutrition, and gives (the body) a bloated feeling and causes gas.

White chickpea is first-degree hot, wet, and heats the body.

The red chickpea and black chickpea are hotter than the white chickpea.

The lentil is first-degree cold, second-degree dry, and could have negative sight effects. The jawsheer and the bird seed both are cold, dry, and then have good effect on the abdominal area.

The broad bean is first-degree cold and dry, causes gas, and is low in quality.

The cumin seed is first-degree hot and second-degree dry, causes anger. Mung (mash) is first-degree cold and wet, and high in quality.

The white, red, and the black beans are hot and wet. All of them are bad for the stomach and cause gas.

The opium poppy is first-degree cold and second-degree dry. (Marginal note: Some people believe it is first-degree hot and soft.)

The sesame (seed) is second-degree hot, wet, and upsets the stomach. The flaxseed (linseed) is a good support for sexual health; it is hot, wet, and soft. The hemp plant seed is second-degree hot and dry, causes headaches. Rice is first-degree hot and second-degree constipating, and highly nutritional.

Chapter two: Regarding types of meat

The meat of lamb and sheep is wet, but lamb meat is wetter. (Marginal note: the meat of sheep and goat is hot and wet; except for the ram, which is cold and dry).

Cow meat is cold and dry.

Suckling calf (fawn) meat is moderate.

Goat meat is cold and dry but kid meat is wetter.

The meat of all the land animals that are born with dark flesh is dry and cold.

---

5 Even if in the original copy the word "fabrics" is not mentioned, in the following pages (Chapter 12) fabric and clothes are discussed.

Rabbit meat is cold and dry.

Pigeon and pullet meat is hot and wet.

The meat of all the chickens and poultry is hot and medium wet.

The meat of the wild bird is hotter, drier, and lighter than the domestic bird. The meat of the sparrow and the partridge is hot and dry.

In comparison with other birds, the meat of water birds is colder, wetter, and heavier. The meat of the domestic birds is harder.

(Marginal note: apart from the other types of bird meat (fowl), the yolk of the chicken egg is hot but the white is cold. Being hot or cold depends on the animal that lays that egg).

Chapter three: Regarding the energy of fish

All fresh fish are cold, wet, and can be digested quickly. Eating fish soothes the stomach and produces sputum.

All salty water fish are hot, dry, and heavy, are not easy to digest, spoil the blood and produce gall and sputum.

The egg of fresh fish is cold, wet, and causes gas and sputum.

Salted fish eggs are hot, heavy, and spoil the blood.

Chapter four: Regarding milk, cream, butter, and cheese (dairy)

Cow milk and sour milk are colder than sheep milk. They are dry and thick. Sheep milk is hotter than goat milk. It is wetter and thicker. Among those three milk types, goat milk is the softest and most delicious. All milk types in general are cold, wet, cause gas, and cool the stomach. Basically, these are considered to be nutritional for tired and nervous people.

Animal fat is hot, soft, strengthens the body, and relaxes the stomach.

Butter is hotter and softer than fat. Fresh cheese is cold, dry, and highly nutritional; but if the cheese is not fresh, then it is hot, dry, and not good for the stomach.

Chapter five: Regarding vegetables

Lettuce is cold, wet, and worth praising for its nutritional value.

The chicory (endive) is very beneficial for the stomach and the liver. It is more likely to be cold and dry.

Watercress is hot and dry, causes headaches, and improves sexual life.

The cress and mustard leaves are hot, dry, cause little gas, and are good for digestion.

The elhamaa elfumah is cold, wet, nutritional, but could have laxative effects.

The batheruuj is hot, wet, and good for the heart and the stomach.

Coriander is cold in general but difficult to digest.

Celery is hot, wet, and good for digestion.

The rue is hot, dry, and good for digestion and releases gas.

Thyme is hot, dry, and good for digestion and keeps the stomach hot.

Mint/elfotenj and elnemmam are all hot, dry, and very good for the stomach.

Tarragon is hot, strong, and difficult to digest.

Sorrel is cold, dry, and good for the abdomen when cooked and drained from its water.

Leek is a hot and dry vegetable that causes headaches, but is good for digestion.

Fenugreek is hot, dry, and causes headaches.

The ek§uuth in general is light and hot. It is a combination of cold and hot and opens the occlusion.

The chard is first-class hot and soothes the constitution.

The sprout, the spinach, and Yemeni beans are cold, wet, and soothing. The "elbelab" soothes the stomach.

The pumpkin (squash) is cold, wet, and soothing.

The eggplant is hot, dry, and spoils the blood.

The asparagus is hot, wet, and improves sexual life.

The kebere is hot, dry, and good for the spleen.

The dill is hot, dry, and not good for the stomach.

Chapter six: The basic energy in other vegetables

The radish is hot, dry, good for digestion and spoils the food.

The onion is hot, wet, very beneficial for digestion and improves sexual life.

The garlic is hot, dry, and very good for the ones who have sputum.

The cabbage is hot, dry, and produces black bile.

The carrot is hot, dry, difficult to digest and produces sputum and causes gas. The mushroom and the truffle are cold, wet, and difficult to digest.

The turnip is hot, wet, easy to digest, and causes gas.

Chapter seven: Benefits of fresh fruit

The sour pomegranate is cold, dry, and suitable for the human constitution. The sweet pomegranate is moderate and the type called "al-emleensy" is delicious and cooling.

The sweet apple is medium hot. The sour apple is cold. Both types are very beneficial for the constitution because they relieve the stomach.

The peach is cold, wet, and thick and produces sputum.

The apricot is cold, wet, and cools (hydrates) the body.

White mulberry is medium cold. The black mulberry is medium hot.

The red mulberry is cold. The red and black are very useful for the constitution, yet the sweet ones are colder and they are more useful for the constitution.

Sweet black grapes are hot, wet, not easily digested, and cause gas. They also soothe the constitution.

White grapes are hotter.

Dates, whether fresh or dry, are hot, wet, cause headaches, but soothe the stomach and strengthen the body.

Dry dates are hot and dry – beneficial for the stomach but not easily digested.

Fresh figs are hot. They are moist according to their tastes. They are suitable for the constitution.

The sweet plum is cold, wet, and good for the abdomen. The sour one is colder and less effective.

The banana is moderate. Its effectiveness depends on its quantity. It is hot and wet.

Sugarcane is hot and wet. It is good when it is moderately consumed. Good for the chest.

The cornelian cherry is cold and dry. Good for the stomach.

The buckthorn is like the cornelian.

The sweet melon is easily digested and transformed to bile. The sour one is cold and easily transformed to sputum.

The gherkin and the cucumber are cold, wet, and produce sputum and cause gas, and their seeds help discharge urine.

Chapter eight: The benefits of dried fruit

The jujube is moderately cold and thins the blood.

The "sebistan" is cold, wet, and soothes the chest.

The almond is hot, soft, and moderate.

Fresh almond is cold, wet, hard, and causes gas.

The pistachio is hot and dry.

The hazelnut is hot, moderately dry, and good for the stomach.

Dried walnut is hot and dry. Fresh walnut is less hot and dry and causes indigestion.

The "boza" (beverage made of slightly fermented millet) is cold, dry, and good for the abdomen.

The dried plum is medium hot and cold and produces sputum.

The energy of dried apricot depends on its degree of sweetness and sourness. The sweet one is more likely to be hot, but the sour one is cold.

The wild pistachio is hot and soft.

The small wild pistachio is medium hot and dry.

Sweet dried grapes are hot and soft. The sour ones are cold and dry.

The wild chestnut is extremely cold and dry.

The chestnut is more moderate than the wild one.

The pine nut (pignolia) is hot and soft.

The fresh Indian walnut is hot and soft, and the dried ones are hot and dry. Sugar is medium hot and soft.

Honey is extremely hot and dry.

Molasses is softer but less hot than honey.

Chapter nine: The benefits of oils

Crude sesame oil is medium in hotness and coldness. The fried kind is hot and dry.

Sweet almond oil is moderately hot but very soft.

"Enfaaq" oil is cold, dry, and causes constipation.

Olive oil is hot and dry.

Violet oil is moderate in hotness and wetness.

The raw rose oil is cold, dry, and causes constipation.

Lily oil is extremely hot and dry.

The dogberry "nasreen" (wild rose) oil is hot and dry.

Willow tree oil is medium in hotness and coldness and causes constipation. Opium poppy oil is hot and anesthetic.

The hemp plant oil is hot and dry.

The water lily "yelnufer" (neylufer) oil is cold and soft or hot and dry. The "ban oil" (willow tree branch oil) is hot and dry.

Mustard oil is hot and dry.

Pistachio oil is hot, soft and the hotness and coldness is moderate. Apple oil is cold and clutching.

Daisy oil is hot and soft.

"Merzijoosh" oil is hot and dry.

Chapter ten: The benefits of fragrant plants

The rose has a compound energy and causes constipation.

The "arad" (lily) is hot and dry.

The daffodil is hot and soft.

The violet is hot and soft.

The "yelnufer" (neylufer) is hot and dry.

The "nemmam" herb[6] is hot and dry.

"Nasreen" herb[7] oil is medium hot.

The "shahisefrem" (a kind of basilicum) in its first stage is medium hot, and when it ripens the seeds become hot and dry.

The "hamahim" (ox tongue) is hot and dry.

The "filinjeshmek" is hot and dry but the hotness is moderate.

The marmajor is hot and dry.

The artemisia and the "khaysuum" (lavender flower) are hot and dry. The "lefah" herb has a compound energy and it is anesthetic.

The willow tree bark is medium hot and cold.

The green jasmine is hot and dry. The white jasmine is moderate, and the yellow jasmine has weak energy.

The "myrtus" herb has a compound energy and it causes constipation.

The daisy chamomile is hot, medium dry and the hotness and the dryness could be extreme.

Chapter eleven: The benefits of fragrances

Musk is very hot and very dry.

Amber is softer than the musk in hotness and in dryness.

The Indian tree is medium hot. It is dry and highly scented and clutching.

The camphor tree's energy is a mixture of dryness and clutching.

The sandalwood tree is medium cold and has a long-lasting distinctive scent.

Saffron is hot and dry.

The "tolan" (El-qaseed) herb is hot and dry.

Carnation is hot and dry.

"Jorbu" is hot and soft.

The "sek" is cold, dry, and conservative.

The "spikes" are medium hot.

The "sennas" is hot and soft.

---

6 It is a small fragrant herb. Its leaves and branches are similar to mint. It is named after its fragrance.

7 It is in many types. One is of Indian origin. It is black, light, and sweet. Another type is of Syrian origin and has a sweet fragrance. The last one is white and has a sweet fragrance, but tastes bitter. It is also called the sea sand.

The "qalqeele" (cardamom) herb is hot and soft.

Chapter twelve: Regarding fabrics

Linen is cold, dry, and clutches energy.

Cotton is medium hot and soft.

Wool is hot and soft.

Camel hair is hot and soft.

The skin of the wild animals is hot and dry.

Beaver's skin and what is similar is cold and dry.

Chapter thirteen: Regarding spices

The coriander herb is medium cold and medium dry.

Cumin is hot and dry.

The kruya (European cumin) is hot and dry.

Wild thyme is hot and dry.

Cinnamon is quite dry and medium hot.

Ginger and the "khawlejan" (galingale) are hot and dry.

Anise is quite hot and dry.

The black cumin is quite hot and dry.

Mustard is quite hot and dry.

The "enjidan"[8] and the roasted "halteeth"[9] are hot and dry.

The "qashim"[10] is medium hot and moist.

Sumac is cold and dry.

The juniper tree fruit is hot and dry.

Salt is hot and dry.

Chapter fourteen: Regarding vinegar, bodha, olives, pickles, and jams

Vinegar is cold and tastes nice.

The bodha is hot and dry.

8 It is called "halteeth" because of the shape of its leaves.

9 Kasni is a type of glue. It is well-known among physicians.

10 A type of herb.

The benefits of the pickles vary as they depend on the ingredients that are used in making them. All the pickles are harmful for the stomach, cause thirstiness, and spoil the blood.

The "big qadhban" tastes nice when it is marinated with vinegar, and it is good for the spleen.

Garlic, marinated with vinegar, especially old vinegar, helps with the digestion and lowers the temperature.

The myrtle tree is low in heat and gas.

The "masinih" is cold and wet.

The "masal" is cold and dry.

The bitter mountain celeriac tastes nice when it is marinated with vinegar, and helps digestion.

The "mensuun" is thicker than the bitter mountain celeriac.

Chapter fifteen: Regarding water, snow, and ice

The best spring water is the one that flows from the top downward through fruitful soil and is exposed to sunshine.

The best rainwater is the water that is gathered in the middle of rocks, exposed to the winds and the sun. Any other rainwater is bad.

According to their nature, snow and ice have no characteristics, but when it snows on a mountain or clear fertile land, then it is pure. Finally, when the ice is formed from fresh water, it looks pure.

Chapter sixteen: Regarding wines

Wine is the best of all fruit juices. It is good for people who have cold constitutions, and good for the hot brain and the hot liver. The hot wine is hot and wet, and when it gets old then it is hot and dry.

The juice of dried grapes is less hot than the wine but causes wind.

Date juice is the softest one among the other juices but it is thick and spoils the blood.

Chapter seventeen: Regarding sherbets and drinks

"Scenjebeen" – plain vinegar and honey sherbet is cold and a good drink. When it is made of roots and seeds, it is hot and it is more useful for the stomach and the liver, because the sherbet of vinegar and honey is sour, and it weakens the stomach and the intestines.

The rose sherbet is medium hot, and it is beneficial when consumed moderately.

The violet sherbet is moderate in both hotness and coldness. It is good for the abdomen and soothes the stomach.

The compound one is good for the stomach and presses the abdomen, and the plain one is good for both.

Apple and quince sherbet is cold and good for the abdomen.

The verjuice is colder than the others. It can cause constipation and relieve thirst.

The pomegranate juice is very useful for the stomach and relaxes the stomach during vomiting.

The mulberry juice is cold so it soothes the constitution. It is good for mouth ulcers and throat aches.

Chapter eighteen: Regarding medicine made from various plants

The "jelincebeen", which is made from sugar, strengthens the stomach and gives heat.

The one made of honey is hotter than the one made from sugar. Marinated violet is moderate in both hotness and coldness and softens the chest and the abdomen.

Marinated ginger heats the body and relaxes the abdomen.

Marinated Indian tree fiber "sheqaqeel" is less effective than the ginger. Marinated "halile/black halile" strengthens the stomach and the whole body. It prevents forgetfulness and takes all the moisture out of the body. Marinated "emlah" is very much like the "halile" but weaker.

Marinated quince and apple strengthens the stomach but causes constipation.

Chapter nineteen: Regarding boiled and fried food

There are many kinds of boiled food. One of these is the "sefeed bagat"; it is soft and causes diarrhea.

The dried "habilat" are strengthening and relaxing, good for the abdomen, and they could be used with spices. They are moderate. The barley, verjuice, pomegranate, sumac juice, and similar juices "keshkiyye" are cooling and cause wind. They all have similar characteristics and energy.

All kinds of fried food are drier than their boiled versions. When sauce is added, they become hotter.

Chapter twenty: Regarding sweets

Sweets are of two kinds. The ones made with honey and the ones made with dough.

The sweets which are made with honey are soft and when consumed they melt in the mouth and help with the digestion. When almond is added, they become difficult to digest and cause bloating.

The sweets made with dough are solid and slow to digest. They block the vessels and joints.

All sweets are very nutritious, increase blood, and support sexual performance.

This is the end of article two.

[24A] The third article

This article is about hygiene, child education, and handling pregnancy. It consists of ten chapters.

Chapter one: This chapter includes sports activities that strengthen the body like wrestling, and less strenuous activities (exercises) like running and walking

There are other personal activities, like reading out loud for oneself, where the head and other organs in the head have to move. These activities heat the organs in the head, clean them, renew their strength (reinforce) and their energies as they nourish them.

Weight lifting, boxing, javelin throwing, and playing with balls, especially with big ones, provide the opportunity to move the body, the neck, the chest, the hands, and the back. These exercises will strengthen these organs, give them energy, and purify them.

Walking fast (jogging) moves the hips, the thighs, the legs, and the feet, so they get energy (heat) and are strengthened. The most balanced sport is slow walking.

Being active (exercising) boosts the natural energy (heat) in the body, whereas, inactivity chills (freezes) and stops the heat and the energy from flowing in the body, which makes the body lose its vitality.

Chapter two: Regarding (steam) bathrooms

The bathroom should be wide, airy, and have plentiful supply of water. Bathrooms should be heated by wood and not by dried cow dung. If heat is supplied through steam in the bathroom, then the materials (the fuel) that are used in heating the water hold utmost importance. If they are good then the steam will be good, but if they are bad, then the steam will also be bad. The heat in the bathroom should not be very high or very low. In the first case, the body will have difficulty in sweating, the heart will become hot, and the heat will cause headaches. In the second case, there will be no steam or sweat.

The water used in the bathroom should be suitable for that specific house. Cold water should not be used in a hot house, and very hot water should not be used in a cold house because these will be the reasons to get (to have) gooseflesh and the clogging of all the pores (breathing points) on the skin. Before getting into the bathtub, a person should stay in the well-ventilated (airy) part of the bathroom for some time.

The body should be in a balanced mood with the water. It is not advisable to stay for a long time in the bathtub, because this will loosen up the body and drain the energy and cause the body to shiver. Upon leaving the bathtub, the face and the head should be wiped with cold water.

After leaving the bathtub and if the body is balanced, water should be poured over the body, because this will give it energy and strength; but with thin and weak bodies, this should not be done. Bathing softens the organs, cleans the body and keeps it fresh and lively (energetic), and removes the residue (dead skin and toxins) from the body.

People who do not do any sports activities should take a bath every day before lunch. They should stay in the bath as long as their strength would allow them to stay.

Taking a bath loosens the humidity in the stomach as it eliminates all the moisture from the stomach and the intestines. It also dries heartburn because it dries the moisture in the body.

Chapter three: Regarding eating and drinking

There are many rules that have to be observed in eating and drinking, such as:

Doing some sports activities before eating.
Relaxing before and after eating.
Doing some sports activities after eating.
Constipated people should eat food that softens their intestines.
People who have diarrhea should eat food that would make them constipated.
During day time, eating should be at the bestbalanced time in terms of weather. In winter eating should be late, and in summer it is preferable to take place during relaxed and comfortable hours.
Food should not be consumed cold in winter or hot in summer.
People should eat a variety (different kinds) of food in season; only one type of food is not good for the body and this is a very important precautionary measure. Not always but mostly the meal should be in different colors. If the dish is oily then either a salty or a spicy (hot) dish must be served next to it. Also, if the dish is salty or spicy then it is good to have an oily dish served with it. If the dish is sour it is obligatory to have a sweet dish next to it. The same should be done with sweet food.

As to incompatible foods, they are the ones that should not be eaten together:

The ones that cause constipation with the ones that cause diarrhea, the ones that are easily digested with the ones that are difficult to digest, the fried with the boiled, fish with meat, dried with fresh, meat with milk, meat with eggs, or fish with legumes.

Drinking water after eating appeases thirst, but the amount of water should not exceed the amount of the meal consumed because it would interfere with digestion, and the water between the stomach and the food particles will make the digestion difficult. The temperature of the water should be adjusted according to the person himself, in a way that should not harm the person or his organs. Warm water is not beneficial.

Chapter four: Regarding sleep and wakefulness

Sleeping relaxes the organs and helps get the food digested and safeguards the constitution and the person. The natural activities in the body develop and mature by sleeping. Excessive sleep (oversleeping) makes the body lethargic (cold), and the person passive and irritable. On the other hand, lack of sleep dries and dehydrates the body, causes fatigue, and hinders (blocks) self-control. Prolonged lack of sleep could lead to madness.

Chapter five: Regarding sexual ability

The need for sex is an innate desire for both adults and elderly people. Yet, the same cannot be said for young children.

If sexual activity is interrupted, it will cause depression and lack of appetite. On the other hand, excessive sexual activity will exhaust the body, weaken eyesight, and damage the brain.

Chapter six: Regarding mental state

Stable happiness strengthens mental health, and, as a result, the person will be productive and full of vitality (energy will comfortably flow in his body).

Grief (sorrow) weakens the psychological state, so the body will be sapped of its strength and drained of its energy.

Extreme anger forces and stirs the heat in the body.

Shyness first stirs the heat in the body and the body starts to sweat, and afterwards this feeling will turn to grief and finally grief will complete the cycle.

Fear is a combination of hope (expectation) and hopelessness (desperation).

Sometimes it spreads heat in the body and sometimes gathers the heat in the in the depth of the body. The first step of anger is rage and its last step is grief, so at the beginning, anger takes its course and at the end, grief completes the cycle. The damage which is done by extreme jealousy is similar to what moderate grief does to the body.

Chapter seven: Regarding the signs of pregnancy and its management

A pregnant woman should avoid the following during the first four months: bleeding herself by cupping (hijamah), having diarrhea, vomiting, intensive fear, loud sounds, food smells, and other intensive odors. If there is a need to have either bleeding by cupping or diarrhea, it would be possible to do so till the end of the seventh month if the woman's constitution is strong enough and not weak or thin. Yet, after that period, the pregnant woman should take care to not do them.

The pregnant woman should protect the mouth of the stomach (esophagus) by avoiding the impulse to eat poor-quality food. Instead of that she could eat rose honey and a mixture of 'iskenjebeen.'

Chapter eight: Regarding lactating mothers and the management of lactation

It is not acceptable for the lactating woman to have any kind of sexual intercourse with her husband in bed while breastfeeding her baby because this kind of action will spoil the milk and make the baby ill. This sort of behavior is completely unacceptable to the Arabs.

During this period, fresh and highly nutritious food should be eaten. The body should not be inactive or calm as this will spoil the milk, and for that reason the mother should do some sports activities (exercises) and keep her body fit.

Chapter nine: Regarding the management of children till puberty

The care that is given to the mother during breastfeeding should be given to the baby as well. When the mother stops breastfeeding her baby, she should give him food. She should start feeding her baby with light and soft food. The food should be given to the baby according to the baby's weight, and this should be done step by step. If the baby's stomach is full, the mother should stop feeding. The child should not be bathed in the bathroom before the age of seven because steam might cause the baby to faint.

Children should not be given wine before they are 14 years old, because wine will weaken (damage) their brains and nervous systems. Children under the age of seven should not be doing tiresome or boring work, or similarly, given tasks that will need disciplinary measures because these will lessen their dynamism and create a barrier for their future education.

Chapter ten: Regarding the management of the human being from the age of 14 till the end of life[11]

The temperament of a person from the age of 14 till the age of 30 is hot and wet. This should be moderate in heat and moisture, so food and nutrition should be moderate in terms of heat and moisture. In case the heat and moisture are in high levels, then food and other related nutrition should be cold and dry.

Starting from the age of 30 till the age of 40, the temperament of the person is hot and dry. The degree of the heat and dryness is moderate. For this reason, food and other nutrition should be in medium heat and dryness. When it exceeds the level of moderation, then the food and other related nutrition should be cold and moist.

The ages between 40 and 60 are cold and dry. If the coldness and the dryness are in their medium levels, then nutrition should also be in medium heat and dryness. When it is above the average, then nutrition and nourishment should be hot and moist.

The ages between 60 till the end of a person's life can take different manners, because during this period the organs are cold, dry, and there is a lot of moist sputum in the cavities of the organs. According to this, a person in any age between 60 and above could be treated relevant to the suitable nourishment mentioned above.

The third article is also finished with the help of Mighty God and His Grace.

11 The age of 14 is considered to be the end of childhood.

[28A] The fourth article

This article is about head illnesses.
It consists of 18 chapters.

Chapter one: Regarding headaches, migraines, and dizziness and hot and cold headaches

The hot headache is the one accompanied with fever and it is divided into two. Either it is caused by blood in the head because the face becomes red, the vessels become swollen, and the pulse becomes high. This can be cured by blood transfusion or cupping "hijamah" or by nutrition such as egg yolk, chicory, and vinegar. Or the headache is because of yellow bile which is distinguished by excruciating pain, fever in the head, the body, and the pulse. This can be cured by consuming the juice of two pomegranates, and as food, a soup made of wheat and "teberzed" sugar with "elhawary" bread and mixed with sour pomegranate and unripe grape juice. The head could be cooled by a compress, which is prepared from rose, juice of "elkhilaf" leaves, a little sandal, camphor, rose flavor, and violet.

The cold headache (without fever) is also divided in two. Either it is caused by love or sadness with symptoms of sleeplessness, talking to oneself, sunken eyes, and a dark-colored face. This can be cured by consuming soup made of black Indian "Ehlilej", dried grapes, cucumbers, crude sugar, oil, and vinegar.

Also the sufferer could inhale violet and lotus oils. A cooked mixture of chamomile, poppy skin, and "elmerzjosh"[12] should be poured over the head. During these days, the person should be eating "Faludej"[13], chicken, and "zirbaj". Or the headache is caused by mildew sputum. The symptoms are: a feeling of heaviness in the head and a feeling of tightness in the face. This can be cured by laxative paste and "shibar" grains and inhaling chamomile, "elmerzjosh", and daffodil. Consuming fowl meat, sparrow and skylark, is also considered to be good. As for the migraine, any of the abovementioned could be applied as treatment. The inhaling should be done from the side where the pain is.

Dizziness can also be treated in the same way. Since repeated vomiting could take place during both migraine and dizziness, the treatment of meals could be interrupted.

---

12 Some say it is saffron.

13 A dessert made from flour and honey.

Chapter two: Regarding the feverish "sersam" illness

The feverish "sersam" illness is caused either from blood or from bile. If it is caused by blood then the symptoms will be: a reddish face, a high pulse, reddish urine, feeling confused, and continuous fever. The cure for this illness is to drink a mixture of barley and jujube juice, and when the patient is not confused, he should be fed with moderate[14] "al hawary" shrimps mixed with "teberzed" sugar. After that and for a couple of days, he should be fed with strained[15] lentil soup[16], almond fat, and vinegar.

If the headache is caused by yellow bile, then the patient's color will be yellow, the tongue will be black, the pulse fast, urine the color of fire, showing severe malaria conditions and raging thirst. The cure for this is sour plums cooked in barley water and drinking squash water mixed with pomegranate juice. When the patient's state of confusion passes, he can be fed with sour pomegranate juice and unripe grape juice and shrimps in honey. After that, the patient should be fed with spinach soup and almond oil.

Chapter three: Regarding the illness of melancholia

This illness is either caused by passionate and hopeless love with fever or without fever. The symptoms for the kind with fever are: a red face, a strong pulse, severe madness, and continuous sleeplessness. It can be cured by inhaling the oil of violet, squash, and opium poppy, drinking breast milk, barley water (juice) with sugar and almond oil. Cold sweet basil water with some drops of handmaiden (jariye) milk and barley water should be poured over the person's head, and the patient could be fed spinach with almond oil.

The symptoms for the kind cold (without fever) are: restriction of urine and a weak and infrequent pulse. The patient should be kept calm. The cure is pouring hot sweet basil water over the patient's head and inhaling sesame oil or "akari"[17] oil and a couple of drops of woman's milk. The patient should drink cooked

14 There is a typo mistake in the Arabic version

15 In the Arabic version, it means peeling while in the translation it means strained.

16 It is translated as soup because doctors prescribe soup to their patients, whereas in the Arabic version it has another meaning.

17 The Arabic word "akari" is a plural word. It means the lower part of the leg, which are the bones underneath the knees. The synonym for the same word means a dish made of animal leg bones, which most probably is the bone marrow.

"efithimon" and eat sliced "faludej" cooked with chicken meat. The patient should take a bath even if he is suffering.

Chapter four: Regarding the epilepsy "Sar'a" illness

If this illness is caused by sputum, then the color of the body will turn to white and the body will tense itself. In this case, the priority is given to the nutrition that provides sputum. It can be cured by grains with fragrance and the "qoqaya". The patient should be fed with wild bird meat either grilled or cooked. The patient should drink the "sekenjebeen" which is the mixture of boiled bird meat and honey and vinegar sherbet. But if the illness shows the signs of "al-sawda" blackness, then the color of the body will be darker and the body will be weaker during the epilepsy; there will be vomiting of sour black bile. In this case the patient is given cooked "Efitheymon", "Agariqun"[18], and "Bayarij Rufus". The patient should have light food and drink plenty of liquid.

Chapter five: Regarding love

If love brings sadness, wakefulness, and loss of weight, then the patient could face insanity. In this case, the patient should be given liquids such as soups to keep his body moist. Also, the patient should eat the sides of the ceruse, take a bath every day, and smell violet oil. This cure is for the body; as for the deep, soul love, then it is one of the psychological illnesses, and the patient is cured with sermons to induce fear or to occupy his mind with other important issues.

Chapter six: Regarding strokes

The sign of a stroke is when the body loses its coordination (releases itself), there is disruption of the senses and nonstop snoring. The patient should take honey syrup until the fourth day. If there is any evidence of fever, then rose water should be given. If the patient recovers on the fourth day, then he should be treated with the stroke medicine, which will be prescribed later with God's will.

---

18 Agariqun originally is a Greek word and is the name of a root. It cures the trees from their poison, is good for constipation, and relaxes the heart. It is also useful for forgetfulness and joint pain.

Chapter seven: Regarding paralysis, numbness, shivering, and wet cramping

The only reason for these illnesses is the irritation as nerves become prolate due to the moisturized sputum. The ones who suffer from this illness have to drink a mixture of honey and spices and eat bread with honey till they regain their strength. When they recover they have to be injected with an expectorant. Later, they should be given laxative pastes and hot seeds.

Chapter eight: Regarding colds

Colds are the moisture that flows out from inside the front of the brain. When the discharged fluid, which comes from the nose, is hot and accompanied by inflammation and fever, then the cure will be bleeding the veins and drinking soft soup from the seeds of "Elisfeed Pache" with salt for a couple of days. Yet, if there is no fever and headache then the best thing is to let the discharged fluid continue to flow nonstop till that part of the brain is cleaned from the discharge. If it is in excess, then, the patient should eat a mixture of sugar, plant leaves, and vinegar heated on a hot stone.

Chapter nine: Regarding eye inflammation

When there is redness because of eye inflammation in the eye accompanied by sweating, in the face, a strong pulse, and redness in the urine, the cure will be bleeding the "Qifal" and cupping the back of the neck. To loosen the bowels, the patient is given a mixture of yellow "Terminalia chebula", bitter cucumber and its seeds. The head should be bandaged with a piece of cloth socked in cold rose water and the feet put in water and massaged. The patient should be fed with food that consists of meat and peeled lentils with almond oil. The bread should be eaten soaked in verjuice and sour pomegranate. When there is less redness in the eye inflammation and more yellow bile is seen, then the cure will be to loosen the bowels by giving the patient yellow "Terminalia chebula" and "sinber" cucumber. There will be no venesection (bleeding) and the food will be the same as above.

But when there is no redness in the eye and only stickiness during the night with crust around the eye (conjunctivitis), then the cure will be drinking "shibeer" seed water, and every night the patient should be given first "eyarij" and then only "fiqra". The patient should take a bath every day. Avoiding dinner, the patient should only be served light and soft food cooked in chickpea water.

Chapter ten: Regarding sight weakness and tear flow

There is no cure for sight weakness during for aging persons and for the elderly. If it happens after a long period of illness or fasting, then the cure will be consuming food of high nutrition to compensate for what the body has lost. In case of eye inflammation or any kind of blow on the eye or falling on the face, the cure will be strengthening the pupils by using "kohl". The recipe for the kohl will be as: one drachma in weight "myrobalan", two drachma in weight "teberzed" sugar, and one drachma Indian tutee.[19]

All these ingredients will be mixed and crushed like powder and from that powder kohl will be made. This kohl prevents tear flow (epiphora) and (agglutination) crust round the eyes, andv it is very beneficial to look at faraway objects every day on an empty stomach; and avoid eating onion, leek, dairy food, and dates. Sexual activity should be avoided too.

Chapter eleven: Regarding ear pain

When ear pain is accompanied with redness, fever in the face, high pulse, redness in the urine, and a feeling of heaviness in the head, the cure will be to bleed the vein from the side where the pain is, and to make the patient have natural diarrhea by giving him yellow melon and "Shanber" cucumber. If these do not work, then the previous recipe can be given again; then cooked nut oil should be poured into the ear. The patient should also consume lentil soup cooked with vinegar, salt, and almond oil. When there is ringing with the ear pain but the pain comes and goes and the pulse is not high and there is no redness in the urine, then the cure will be to let the patient drink "shibar" seed drink "shibar" seed to purify the stomach and the brain. Also, make the patient vomit (throw up) and gargle. Easily digested food should be given such as "zarbajat" cooked in oil. Marjoram leaves cooked in oil can be poured into the ear.

When there is some discharge coming from the ear following the pain as a result of a rupture, the suppurated discharge should not be stopped from leaking until it eventually ceases. If the discharge continues, the reason could be what the patient had consumed; in which case, the patient should take a bath and the affected ear should be treated with an ear wick (swab) made from a piece of cloth soaked in rose water and sprinkled with camphor.

19 It is the name of a stone from which "kohl" is made.

Chapter twelve: Regarding nose pain

One of the kinds of nose pain is when there is a stinky smell coming from the nostrils. The cure for this pain is to purify the patient's stomach by vomiting, and then purify the intestines for a number of times with the help of a laxative paste that is made of "shibar" seeds and "eyarij" seeds. If the patient could bear (endure) it, he could gargle with a mixture made of crushed wild thyme and mustard mixed with wine or honey juice or vinegar to purify the nasal passage. During the night, the patient could have a nice-smelling spice seed in his mouth. The same thing could be added to a fresh-smelling liquid to be inhaled. The patient should avoid dinner and eating heavy meals.

The other kind is nose bleeding. When bleeding takes place it means that the body is full of blood. For that reason, it is necessary to bleed the head veins from the side where the nose is bleeding. If this process stops the bleeding, then there is no need to do anything else. Yet if it is not enough, then cupping should follow. If there is no change in the patient's situation, then the liver should be cooled with a piece of cloth soaked in a mixture of sandalwood, rose water, and grained rose and camphor. It is also useful to make the patient sneeze by making him breathe "saduran" water and camphor or what is called as lamb tongue with bean water and camphor, and also by preparing a wick and soaking it in a mixture of gallnut water and grained "qalqitar" and putting it inside the nostrils (nose holes). It is good to pour cold water over the head from a pitcher. The other kind is the weakness of smell. The cure for this is to make the patient inhale the vapor of cooked land and river pennyroyal with sesame.

Chapter thirteen: Regarding lip cracks

There is a very beneficial balm for lip cracks, which is made of duck's inner fat, white wax, and violet oil. First, melt the wax and the fat together, then keep aside to get cold, then many things like kohl or ground starch could be sprinkled over the mixture; and after mixing all these ingredients, it could be used.

Chapter fourteen: Regarding teeth, gums, and molar teeth pain

First, identify the location of the pain. If the pain is in the gums, the flesh will be swollen and red. Sometimes it is accompanied with blood. The cure for this is the cupping from the cavity of the back of the neck. If it is still not enough, blood should be taken from the head veins. The mouth should be either washed with "feraj" water or with a mixture made of sumac and dried "kasphara" herb, and cold food should be consumed. When the teeth are healthy, but the pain is in the roots of the teeth with swelling, then the swelling should be identified. If the swelling is filled with substance like blood or bile, then blood should be taken from the vein. The patient should be given a mixture of yellow "myrobalan" herb and "shanber" cucumber to drink.

If the swelling is caused by sputum or black bile, the patient should drink a mixture of "eyarij" or "ebluuj" seeds, or "quqayi" or "istenhiqun" seeds. If the swelling is not clear, the patient should wash his mouth a couple of times with *Citrullus colocynthis* peel cooked in sesame oil and a little "Agir". Easily digested food is recommended, and it is preferable to wash the mouth with hot gum oil for a couple of times. If there is tooth decay and the pain is due to the decay, then the patient should drink a mixture of gum oil and poppy skin and Roman "filuniye" peel. In the case of molar teeth, the cure will be to bite hot cooked egg yolk and to rub the teeth with hot oil, and eat hot fatty meat.

Chapter fifteen: Regarding mouth and teeth blisters

If the blisters are red, the cure for this is cupping from the cavity of the back of the neck, and gargling. Also it is beneficial to drink "taub" syrup, verjuice and "ribyas" syrup, and chew grape branches, or bite fresh almond crust and eat sweet and dried grape cooked in almond oil and sugar. The patient can also eat barley soup or lentil soup cooked in almond oil. In addition to the above, the patient can chew purslane.

If the blisters have white pus, the area should be rubbed with sugar powder and a bit of green "ziraj". The patient should apply ground yellow myrobalan on the teeth several times. It is also beneficial to wash the mouth with yellow myrobalan.

If the blisters have black pus, the area should be covered with ground yellow arsenic or ground marble or ground "al qalqtar". After an hour, if the blackness is still present, the treatment should be applied again till the area is reddish, and when it becomes red, the area should be cleaned. Then the patient should gargle with almond oil and apply, on that specific area, ground "haba" and ground "asa". For a couple of days the patient should consume only boiled egg and egg soup.

Chapter sixteen: Regarding polishing the teeth and freshening up the mouth

The best way to make the teeth white and shiny and polished, and keep the mouth fresh and smelling good is by dipping the finger into honey first and then into the "taberzed" sugar and using the mixture to polish the teeth. Using hot "siyunat" every day can harm the gums and their flexibility, but at the same time purify the saliva in the mouth.

As to freshening up the mouth, it is preferable to gargle every day of the week with a mixture of honey, vinegar, salt, and water, but it is not advisable to exceed the usage of this solution.

Chapter seventeen: Regarding the uvula, the tonsils, and diphtheria

When swelling takes place in the uvula and the tonsils, which are on both sides of the throat and at the starting point of the ears, this will affect the muscles around the throat or the ones at the beginning of the gorge and the gullet. As a result, the patient will suffer from breathlessness. If this situation continues, and it is impossible to get into normal breathing again, accompanied by fever and tenseness in the body, then, the best thing to do is to immediately bleed one of the elbow veins. Following this and up to the third day, the patient should gargle with a juice made of pomegranate crushed with its seeds and peel or a mixture of boiled pomegranate blossom, sumac, and rose.

After urination the patient will relax. If the throat path is open, the patient should consume boiled "shibar" cucumber and gargle with fig juice. For the saliva, gargling with a mixture of plantago seeds, white quartz seeds, and white sugar could be beneficial; as well as consuming egg yolk.

When the throat is not swollen and there is no difficulty in swallowing, the patient should be injected with a mixture of fruit juice, cooked marshmallow, and red sugar.

If the cause comes from sputum, moisture, and milking, then blood should not be taken; gargling with fresh walnut juice will suffice. When the throat path is clear, the easiest cure is to inject the patient with a mixture of cooked "shanber" cucumber, and yellow and black myrobalan.

When the throat path is not clear, the patient should be injected with a strong shot till he feels better; and on the third day, he should gargle with a mixture of fig juice and licorice. When the swelling diverges and a discharge occurs, the patient should be served plain raisin juice or plain honey juice. If it stops, then blow into his throat.

Chapter eighteen: Regarding the comment that occurs in the throat

When sticky sputum (mucus, saliva) occurs in the throat, and it is clearly seen, then you can pull it out with nippers. If the eye is not capable of seeing it, try to make the patient drink wormwood soaked in water, which will kill the comment. The patient should drink daffodil water, lubinus water, or hot thick vinegar.

The end of article four.

[36A] The fifth article

The fifth article is about throat illnesses and it consists of four chapters.

Chapter one: Regarding coughing, catarrh, and pleurisy

If the coughing is dry with little saliva, with no visible signs of illness in the body, but the cough is accompanied with fever and the color of urine is not good, then the patient should drink plantago seeds' juice and violet juice. Also the patient should drink barley water with violet juice. He should be given soups and light meals, such as spinach cooked in almond oil. Yet if there is no evidence of fever, the patient should eat the fresh and soft parts of the meat and the fish. The chest should be rubbed with a mixture of violet oil, wax, and pumpkin water.

When coughing is accompanied with sputum (saliva) and the body shows illness and the cold originates from the head, then bleeding should take place. After that, the patient should drink a mixture of barley water marinated with violet, and eat the abovementioned food.

If coughing is dry with no saliva and no fever and the body shows no sign of illness, then the patient should drink "shanber" cucumber with white sugar cooked with maidenhair, and eat chickpeas and a mixture of broad beans and almond oil. If coughing is preventing the patient from sleeping, then he should be given plain opium poppy juice.

Chapter two: Regarding asthma

When a person feels severe imbalance in his movements while working accompanied with shortness of breath and heaviness in the chest, then he should eat cooked dry hyssop herb and drink a mixture of island onion, keven tree thorn, and yellow figs; and with this mixture, the patient should eat peeled almond with honey, caraway, and dill; and drink distilled hot water.

Chapter three: Regarding palpitations

If the palpitation is covering the whole body and the pulse is high, then blood should be taken from the left basilic vein. The patient should drink camphor tablets melted in plain apple juice. When the body temperature is normal, the patient should drink *Terminalia chebula* with plain honey and vinegar; and eat chicken cooked in verjuice; and keep the chest cool by using a piece of cloth soaked in rose water, camphor, and sandalwood every day. If there is some evidence of coldness accompanying the palpitations, then the patient should take amber medicine and sweet musk with stimulants and drink lily juice. If the illness continues, the patient should drink “shibar” seeds and take musk medicine and eat cooked chicken (bird) soup. It is useful to rub the patient’s chest with lily oil and yellow wax. In addition, the patient should inhale fragrant vaporized odors and eat chicken and bird meat. If the palpitations continue after the illness with severe vomiting, then the patient should eat blood-forming food and drink wine and avoid sexual activity.

Chapter four: Regarding blood in the saliva

If foamy, rose-colored blood is seen while coughing, the patient should be given “Elber” tablets with chicken soup. If the color of blood is reddish and there is no foam, then the patient should have amber tablets and pomegranate rose tablets and a mixture of plantago juice, marshmallow, chalk, pomegranate rose, and the seeds of plantain. In addition, he should drink the mixture of verjuice and vinegar. Then, the chest should be bandaged with the following mixture: “kender”, coral, “qaqya” wax, and rose oil. The patient should drink plenty of soups consisting of lentils, verjuice, sumac juice, and “enqaq” oil or almond oil marinated in Armenian clay and chalk water.

This is the end of article five.

[37B] The sixth article

This article is about abdominal illnesses and their relations to food and nutrition.
There are 14 chapters.

Chapter one: Regarding stomach weaknesses

When the food is not digested properly, you have to look for the reason behind it. Is it from the stomach, or from mixing up food, or only from cold. If it is from cold, the cure will be only to keep it warm. To do this, crush and sieve a mixture of long pepper, ginger, oat bread, and *Pistacia lentiscus*, then mix it with filtered honey. The patient should take seven drachma with water, especially with cold water, dose after dose. He should also eat food cooked with bird meat.

If, in addition to the cold, the stomach is facing other symptoms, then the patient should eat a mixture of soup which is made of meat and a lot of dill mixed with water and marinated with honey, mustard, and radish; then wait for one hour till the food spreads around and cuts the sputum. After that, he can drink a lot of liquids from honey and vinegar, but with hot water; or can eat soup made of red beans, white salt, and dill with some drops of oil. The patient should eat this mixture and vomit till the stomach is cleaned; and when the stomach is cleaned, the previously prescribed paste should be taken. This will be enough for the patient, with the will of God. If the patient dislikes vomiting or he finds it difficult, then every night he should drink one whit (lump) of dill till his stomach is cleaned.

Chapter two: Regarding nausea

If the nausea happened after eating a meal, then the cause is the meal itself, which should be vomited; after that, the patient should drink water. Yet if the nausea happened before the meal with signs of yellow bile, then the patient should drink cold or fizzy water and should force himself to let the yellow bile come out of the upper part of the stomach. After that, the patient should drink plain pomegranate juice. If the yellow bile signs are not clear, then he should drink pomegranate juice with mint, which will be enough to heal the stomach.

Chapter three: Regarding colic

If the colic happens immediately after eating, the cure will be to vomit, especially if the pain is in the stomach. If the pain is in the navel, it should be rubbed with a mixture of lily oil, a little of powder of musk and "elgaliye", and compressed with a stupe (bandage). The mixture could also be cooked as mash so that the navel will loosen and gas will find its way out from the bottom. The intestine could be cleaned with a mixture made of anise butter mixed with cumin and hot water and sugar; or hot juice mixed with a little pepper and ginger powder, which will be a cure drink for the intestine. Yet if there is some kind of severe stinging (biting), fragmentation in the abdominal cavity, and burnout in the back part of the abdomen, then this is because of the bitterness (soreness) of the gall. The cure for this is a hot soup with some drops of almond, rose, or violet oil with which the patient can defecate and get rid of the soreness.

Chapter four: Regarding hiccups

If the hiccups occur after eating and the food comes from the stomach to the mouth, the best thing to do is to throw up. If the patient hates vomiting or cannot vomit, then he should suck a mixture of quince, sweet pomegranate and mint, or pennyroyal, or "elnemmam". If the hiccups happen after vomiting, then let the patient drink almond oil. If it happens for any other reason especially like mixing food types or eating something rotten (spoiled), which could be a reason for the indigestion, then the patient should drink "al shibar" seeds and "al ayarij" seeds. He should also eat easily digested food or drink vinegar and honey to strengthen the stomach; or drink terminalia, which relaxes mild hiccups; or the patient should be given extraordinary news to confuse and distract his mind, making him forget about the hiccups. There is another way to overcome hiccups and that is to hold your breath or hold your nose and do not breathe for a while till the breath returns back to the abdomen.

Chapter five: Regarding diarrhea

The cause of diarrhea is excess in eating. The stomach starts to digest the food up to its capacity then stops digesting, so, although some of the food stays half digested, it is still naturally pushed out of the stomach. This action mostly causes the upper part of the stomach and the canals that are connected to the intestines to swell. Also, it could give bitterness to the sputum, and afterwards, this reaction will turn to diarrhea. The person who has diarrhea should allow the indigestible food to go out, if the body is weak and the diarrhea will not stop; the body will clean itself by throwing out all the indigested food. During this period, the patient should not eat anything. If he is not capable of doing this, he can eat some bread with cooked food or eat the food which hurts him less. When the diarrhea stops, yet the pain is still there, then for a few days, the patient should eat light food. But if the diarrhea gets worse and the excrement is in different colors, yet there is no pain or feeling of fragmentation inside, and it has been a while since the patient had taken any laxatives, if he holds the strength, he should defecate.

But if there is the feeling of fragmentation inside and pain and the body starts to lose strength, then the following things should be taken into consideration: if the color of the excrement is yellow and the person feels thirsty but there is no abdominal noise or gas, then eating a mixture of cow milk and crushed bagel is enough. If another cure (medicine) is required, then the patient should drink a mixture of baked plantain soaked in sumac water and rose water. Yet if the internal pain and the feeling of fragmentation increase, the patient should drink egg yolk blended with rose oil. If only the diarrhea is left with no pain, then the patient should eat the "Sikbaj" which is cow meat cooked in vinegar with an addition of bread crumbs and should drink cold water. If the excrement is wet accompanied with noisy gas from the abdomen but there is no feeling of being thirsty or any epigastric burning, then the patient should drink a mixture of two drachma of garlic paste (butter), half drachma mastic gum, blended with myrtle extract and should eat a mixture of dried black grape, basil, walnut oil, olive oil, and mustard foam cooked in melilotus water.

When the patient is constipated, he should repeat the same food for a few days to get back to normal. If diarrhea is accompanied with blood, then the same cure (medicine) should be used; in addition to that, the patient can drink a mixture of roasted (baked) plantago and purslane seed and two drachma from both should be added to clay, a drachma of Arab gum, and the chalk, and all of these will be blended and given to the patient to drink altogether once. The patient can drink plantago and purslane juice as well. As for nutrition, he can drink verjuice or sour pomegranate juice or eat bagel soaked in pomegranate seed juice.

Chapter six: Regarding dysentery

If the patient is complaining of frequent pain in the abdominal area and the excrement is a bit foamy with sputum, then he has dysentery. Sometimes blood can be seen. The cure for this will be drinking a mixture of watercress butter and lily oil and eating a mixture of walnut, aisin, pigmentis oil, and mustard mousse with bread. Yet, if there is blood then the patient should drink fried "Hashfere" powder mixed with water and rose oil.

Also, he should eat cooked egg yolk with bread or walnut with bread. When the disease is severe, then the bowel gets out of the anus (prolapsus). To cure this, the patient should take some from each of the following: pomegranate rose, ashes, and bitter Lathan leaves, which he should crush, sieve, and puddle with water.

Then he can eat it with nasreen oil. If there is blood with the dysentery, then the patient will take some from each of the following: pomegranate blossom, ashes, and burnt seashells, which he should crush, sieve, and puddle with plantain juice. If not, the patient will take one of the mentioned ingredients with rose water (juice) and rose oil.

Chapter seven: Regarding gripes

Gripes are either caused by chilling the intestines and becoming sticky, or because of inflammation and thick gases (winds) which cause pain due to stretching; and a third reason could be due to the twisting or drying of the intestines. The cure for these types could be the following: first, when the patient feels the pain, he should not immediately take hot or diarrhea medicines, especially if he has recently eaten something. This will increase his pain and lead to other symptoms. The patient should not eat till the pain ceases (passes), and he should sip hot water. He should avoid eating for at least two days. If the patient is physically weak and cannot avoid eating, then he should have cooked meat with spices and a piece of soft bread (crumbs). He should also drink two drachma of natural laxative pastes and wait for four hours, then he can eat the following: 10 drachma each of celery root bark and fennel root bark, adding to the mentioned ingredients a mixture of two drachma of celery seed and cumin and the whole lot cooked in a pound of water. The mixture should be boiled till one third is left, then strained, and seven drachma of "shanber" cucumber and ten drachma of cheese sugar should be added to it and the whole lot should be boiled. This mixture should be drunk hot. If there are signs of fever, or there is fever, then the patient should take one and a half drachma of castor oil mixed with four drachma of fresh vinegar oil.

If the patient is cured and there is no more pain, then he should eat a mixture of fatty quail, chickpeas, dill, cumin, and oil solution. If an injection is needed as part of the treatment, then first, one third of a pound of fresh thorn should be boiled and one ounce of oil solution or about 20 drachma of red sugar and one whit of powder dough salt should be added to it and, with the will of God, if the patient needs to get completely cured, then he also has to take a mixture of honey molasses and cow gall in oil solution one by one.

Chapter eight: Regarding abdominal worms

The best thing which reduces the occurrence of the abdominal worms is to eat a mixture of "elfornj" with vinegar and water on an empty stomach or to eat lupine on an empty stomach. As for a medicine to cure it, the patient should drink one of the following or as a mixture drink "al-shaykh al-armeni" or a mixture of seeds of Indian sunflower, Kabul rice, and absinthe separately or together.

Chapter nine: Regarding liver pains

When the pain in the liver starts all of a sudden and it is accompanied with visible fever and extreme thirst with high pulse and redness in the urine, then the right basilica vein should be bled. The liver should be cooled with a piece of cloth soaked in the following mixture: rose water, sandalwood, camphor, cold (with ice) "al khilaph" leaf juice, or quince and apple juice. The patient should drink a mixture of barley water with plain honey and vinegar or sour pomegranate juice. If the patient has no fever then he could eat a mixture of chicken cooked in verjuice with squash and purslane, but if there is fever then only verjuice without the chicken. Also, the patient has to drink chicory with honey and vinegar for two or three days.

When the pain comes consecutively accompanied with paleness, irritation on the face, some feeling of thirst, but the coldness and the moisture is clear, then every day the patient should drink one of the medicines, which contain curcuma and rose water about one whit with seed root juice liquids and should eat sparrows and wild birds.

Yet, if the urine consists of different colors, especially red accompanied with fever, then the patient should drink the following mixture on the same day till his temperature becomes normal: chicory, ivy, gooseberry, husk tomato, fennel with one third ounce of concentrated vinegar, and honey. The patient should also eat *Berberis vulgaris* cooked in oil solution with honey. If the fever becomes higher, then the pastes should be used again and the liver should be covered with a bandage soaked in seed water. Another paste that could be used for the same situation is a mixture of: laudanum, mastic, saffron, Indian hyacinth, and black algae. A piece of each item should be taken, ground, and then kneaded with licorice oil and mastic melted in yellow wax. After applying this paste on the liver, it should be covered with a piece of cotton cloth soaked in boiled "eljilq" seed water. When some signs of swellings are seen clearly on the liver, the bandaging should be repeated.

Chapter ten: Regarding spleen pains

When spleen pain is accompanied with visible fever, and colored urine with high pulse, then the main vein or the left axillary vein should be bled. The patient should drink a mixture of green leaf juice, chicory leaves juice, mixed with the "al kabara" root, weeds, and vinegar and honey. He could also eat food cooked with bird meat or goat meat. If the pain makes the patient's skin color greenish black, with weak stomach, and poor digestion accompanied with noises in the stomach and a lot of winds (gas), then the patient should drink what weighs two drachma of light laxative combined with almond and *Agaricus bisporus*, one weight of barley and wheat. This mixture should be drunk every night. The patient should also eat food cooked with wild bird meat once in the day and at night. He should also eat well-cooked food, but if he does not like to eat it, he should eat figs, almond, and Khurasan grapes and pistachio. He should only drink hot water. The spleen should be bandaged with the following paste: take one part of both yellow mud and blue resin, add to it vinegar, and keep it for one day and a night, then put the whole lot into the mortar, beat it till it is stewed.

After that, melt one ounce of duck fat and one of chicken fat after removing all the veins and the skin. Add the mixture to the one in the mortar. On top of it add two drachma from each of the following: the medulla of the cow leg and lichen, "fuqah al adkhar", saffron, and spikes, till the whole mixture becomes a powder, then cook it and put the mixture on a piece of cloth and put it on the spleen. Then take another piece of cloth soaked in lily oil and bandage it tightly on the forehead at the beginning of the day and before eating for four hours, then take the piece of cloth off and let the patient take a shower and clean the area with a mixture of cooked ruta, *Tamarix aphylla* leaves, and herbs.

Chapter eleven: Regarding jaundice

If the patient's pupils and the whole body is pale (yellowish), especially if it is accompanied with fever, then this distemper is due to jaundice. When the fever is gone, the body will get its relief. The cure for this fever is the same as the cure for the jaundice. Yet, if the patient is suffering from real jaundice with some fever, then the cure for this will be: chicory juice, "yanj" rice with vinegar and honey. It is also advisable to take a bath before eating every day. Also to run the intestine, the patient should eat the following mixture: the yellow terminalia, chebula, "shanber" cucumber, and the "taberzed" sugar. If yellowness is absent in the iris, then the patient should inhale some drops of vinegar mixed with rose oil. He should eat meat cooked in vinegar – preferably, very sour cow meat and stinging nettle. When there are no visible signs of fever with jaundice, but it all happened after a heavy meal or syrupy food, then let the patient have two drachma of "aft" seed every night, and make him eat only light food; the sour ones cooked in solution oil will be better.

Chapter twelve: Regarding kidney pains

If a sudden pain appears in the kidneys after excessive consumption of meat and dessert or wine and if this is accompanied with a high pulse and redness in the urine, the patient should be bled on the side where the pain is from the basilica vein, and given light food like spinach, squash, egg yolk, peeled Indian peas, peeled lentils, and almond oil. For lunch, he should drink a mixture of watermelon and cucumber seeds, wild cucumber, peeled squash mixed with white poppy seeds, and chalk, all of which must be mixed with violet syrup. If this is not enough, then the patient needs to drink a mixture of fruit juice and raw rose oil mixed with rose water. If the patient did not have any sexual activities for a period of time, let him do so and if he feels extreme thirst, then give him cooked barley water mixed with squash. He can also drink bagel in cow buttermilk and eat soft fish cooked with vinegar, spices, and onion or chicken in verjuice or eat a mixture of Sind watermelon with cucumber mixed with barley juice or mixture chilled in snow. The area where the kidney pain is can be rubbed with a paste made of rose water, sandal, camphor mixed with portulaca, squash, or cucumber juice.

If the pain comes suddenly, but there was no continuous pain, and blood does not stop, then let the patient drink a mixture of dragon blood tree, clay, olibanum, poppy, and Arab glue, a drachma of each mixed with portulaca juice; and the patient should eat sour lentils. If there is severe pain in the kidneys accompanied with sand in his urine flask, then that is due to the gravel in the kidney. In this case, the patient should drink one of these medicines: peeled watermelon seeds, ground grape seeds, or celery and anise or drink a mixture of one drachma of crushed "yanj" rice seeds and thorn core seeds, mallow seeds, mulukhiye seeds, rose, mixed with fresh sour liquids. He should also eat black chickpeas with almond oil and avoid dairy products and heavy meals.

If the patient is suffering from kidney weakness and facing some symptoms of cold, then he should drink Galen every day to warm the kidney and the bladder. He should also consume "faniz" syrup, which is made by boiling sugarcane, and eat chicken or birds which are kept in water and salt solution first and then cooked in olive oil. For the dessert, a light meal with honey and plain oil will be enough. The patient should inhale nice fragrances like jasmine and drink wine. He should avoid bathing.

Chapter thirteen: Regarding bladder diseases

If gallstones are found in the bladder, which is in general seen in boys, the symptoms will be as follows: white urine accompanied with white sand particles and continuous itching in the penis. The patient, according to his age and strength, should be given mallows to drink and eat cooked one sixth of a drachma of "elnanukhe" and the "faniz". He can also drink the amount of one sixth of a drachma to one drachma of celery seed powder mixed with honey juice, and eat radish and carrot cooked in either oil solution or walnut oil. If there is dripping of urine or burning yellow urine, or there are some signs of fever, then make the patient drink cold seeds in violet juice, which we had mentioned previously. The patient could also drink bagel in cow buttermilk, and eat spinach cooked in almond oil. When burning in the urine is intense, the patient should drink milk yogurt with sugar and relieve the pain by using a combination of dairy products. If there is no pain or burning with the dripping or stinging and the color of the urine is white but cold and moisture is clear, then the patient should drink quince juice with Galen paste and hot seeds with honey. He can also drink ripe wine and the mixture of *Origanum minutiflorum* and menyanthes, and eat bread with honey and walnut.

Chapter fourteen: Regarding anus diseases

When pain occurs in the anus and gets worse and constipation takes place, then it means that there is some kind of swelling in that specific area. The patient should sit on warm water mixed with the following ingredients: marshmallow leaves, "milukhiyah", and pieces of squash with its seeds cooked together. After that the area should be rubbed with almond oil mixed with rose water and could be loosened with a mixture of "shanber" cucumber, grape juice, and "faniz" syrup. Yet if the patient is still facing difficulty, then bleeding should be done from the basilica. He should eat egg yolk blend with linseed and "portulaca" (water broad bean) cooked in almond oil.

If there is bleeding in the anus and it is continuing and the anus area is not healthy, then the patient should be treated by either amber tablets or lotus tablets. When there is no fever, then olibanum seeds cooked with trotters and vegetables will be good. But if the bleeding is extreme, the patient should be injected with crushed Myrtus communis water mixed with pomegranate blossom or the pomegranate blossom could be mixed with mastic oil.

This is the end of article six.

[46A] The seventh article

This article is about genital organs.
It consists of six chapters.[20]

Chapter one: Regarding penis diseases

Sometimes gases that could accumulate in the penis due to the heat and moisture could make the penis tense and erect without having any sexual activity. In this case, first, make the patient vomit several times after eating. Second, the patient should rub the pubes with a mixture of Armenian clay and vinegar and bandage the area aligned to the pubes with a mixture of soaked plantain seeds mixed with portulaca (water broad beans) water. He should also drink ruta graveoleus seeds and "al phinkhasq" seeds with cold water and eat colorful plant seeds cooked in almond oil.

Chapter two: Regarding the appearance of pre-seminal fluid and prostatic secretion

These two fluids appear either after a sexual activity and the need to have such an action, or after loosening in the semen producing organs, or from the intensity (severity) of the semen. The cure for the first one is to practice the sexual activity. For the second one, the usage of meryanthes paste with sage; and for the third one, the patient should drink a mixture of cold seeds with stimmed milk, rusk and portulaca (water broad beans).

Chapter three: Regarding testicular diseases

When there is hot swelling in the testicles, then bleeding should be done from the basilica and rub a mixture of sandalwood with rose mixed with rose water on the swelling. The patient should eat plenty of nuts. If there is increase in fever and the swelling stiffens, then the area should be bandaged with a paste made of broad bean powder, and grilled meat with kidney oil.

20 The original copy mentions seven chapters, whereas, here it is only six chapters.

Chapter four: Regarding hernia

Hernia occurs for two reasons, either due to the fall of the intestines or because of the dripping in the testicles. The patient should avoid all kinds of food or drink that cause gasses. He should drink liquids which contain garlic or calf churn. In addition, the wind (gas) path should be blocked with a piece of plaster.

Chapter five: Regarding womb diseases

If the woman's menstruation is extreme and her breasts are full, then bleeding should be done from the basilica. When the color of the menstrual blood is white, yellow, or black, then the intestines should be softened with "elesmetikhaqun" seed and the patient should eat lentils and dairy products. She should also sit on a mixture that consists of cooked and pressed olive residues with pomegranate peels and in the spring, she can use grape juice, instead. If the menstrual flow does not occur when the woman is not pregnant or of old age and the body is swollen, then there should be bleeding from the leg.

The patient should drink cooked terminalia and madder and eat a mixture of cooked fenugreek and cooked onion and leek.

Chapter six: Regarding sexual intercourse

If the person is driven away from sexual activities, and is not that much interested or passionate and eats very little, then he should drink fatty hot buttermilk or milk with sugar and ginger. He should avoid bitter wines. Also, the waist should be rubbed with violet oil or lotus oil. The patient should eat fresh and soft fish. If the patient is of cold nature, then he should eat marinated ginger, eggs, and pepper. He can also eat vegetables with honey, onion, and fatty chickens and birds and can drink aged (old) wine. It is preferable to rub the waist with jasmine oil and other precious fragrances.

This is the end of article seven.

[47A] The eighth article

This article is about gout disease, sciatica, and joint pains.
The origins of the abovementioned diseases are all the same, but they have different names due to their locations. If one of the feet's joints is affected, then it is called gout; and if the hip area is affected, then it is called either hip pain or sciatica. Also if the joints are affected, then it is called joint pain, but if this pain is located in the joints of the back bones, then it is called back pain.

If there is some indication of fever, high pulse, and redness or dark yellowness in the urine, then bleeding should take place from that specific area. The patient should drink cooked terminalia and colchicum and bandage the joints of the thump with a mixture of plantago seeds soaked in vinegar and mixed with rose water. Food restrictions should be applied to the patient and he should eat light meals. The best will be eating nuts marinated in fresh oil solution till the pain is relieved. If there is no pain, the patient can eat grouse.

When the pain is severe with clear symptoms, the patient should vomit for couple of times, and then he should drink the "al stamkhiqoun" seed juice or be injected with a mixture of hot oils and ripe boiled bone water. He should be made to suffer hunger and only eat once a day for two days. When the pain is gone, he can eat chicken and wild birds, but he should not drink wine or have heavy meals; and he should also abstain from any sexual activity.

***The end of* article eight.**

[47B] The ninth article

This article is about illnesses that occur on the skin related to drawing blood and hijamah.

Chapter one: Regarding hair diseases

When there is a disease in head hair and beard and moustache hair, the patient should clean his stomach by vomiting. Then he should examine his body to see if it is swollen with high pulse. In addition, if urine is red or dark yellow, then bleeding should take place till he feels better; and he should also use laxative seeds. He should eat pure white bread and avoid dairy products, fruit, autumn vegetables, and salty food. He should also abstain from any sexual activities. When blood symptoms are not visible, then there is no need for the bleeding, and the patient should continue with what we had advised previously.

When the lichen and the trichoschisis are spreading then the cure will be purifying the head and the body as we explained above. If there is dryness in the hair, then shaving will be enough along with washing the head with a mixture of hollyhock, borax, and terminalia leaves. To get rid of the lichen permanently, the patient should snuff every night if he is capable of doing it.

Chapter two: Regarding clearing the face from spots and freckles

When the spots and freckles increase in number, the cure will be bleeding. Yet if the body is swollen, the patient should drink a mixture of cooked *Agaricus bisporus* and *Cuscuta epithymum.*

He should apply a paste made of watercress seeds on the skin till it heals and should eat light food. When the ulcers are healed and only some trails are left, then these trails could be cured by applying the following mixture: almond oil and wax. When the trails improve the patient can eat his/her normal food.

Chapter three: Regarding herpes and fungal diseases

To cure these diseases, we should start purifying the body by bleeding it and feeding the patient with cooked terminalia and healthy food. The second thing is to prepare the following medicine to be applied on the specific area: the essence of yellow terminalia seeds, the Kabuli and licorice leaves. The powder obtained from these ingredients should be mixed with vinegar, oil, and wax, and be applied on the affected area. The patient should be given light food.

Chapter four: Regarding the whiteness of the skin (vitiligo)

If it is very new and has not spread around, then the first thing to do will be: if the skin is white, the patient should vomit by using the white hellebores; and if the skin is black, then he has to use the black hellebores as a laxative; or only purifying the body with laxatives will be enough. Whereas, with the white using the Galen as laxative will be good.

When the skin is black then bleeding is useful. Also, the cooked cuscuta will act as laxative. The patient should have light food, and he should have daily baths before breakfast, except when using the medicine. The body should be rubbed with pepper and honey.

Chapter five: Regarding itching

The best way to stop the itching is to use the following as laxative every day to clean the body: seeds of *Agave americana*, terminalia, roses, and mastic. But when the body is swollen, bleeding should take place and the body should be slowly purified with laxatives. When the veins are cleaned, the patient should continue to take baths and rub his body with green glasswort until the skin is cured. The food should be light and consist of meat and pure bread; the patient should avoid wine and sexual activities.

Chapter six: Regarding measles, small pox, urticaria, and impetigo

When the fever and blisters show smallpox and measles, the cure will be quinine. The patient should drink barley water and eat peeled lentils. He should also drink a mixture of "al amleesi" pomegranate juice and rose oil. The patient should have drops of rose water into the eyes at the medial side. If the nature of the bowels is smooth (bowels are soft), then the patient should be given barley soup and fried lentils and he can drink fruit juices. Yet, if the blisters have ripened, then the patient should inhale the mixture of tamarisk and rose petals, and rose and myrtle powder should be spread all over the bed. When the fever is gone and there is constipation, then he should be given chicken cooked in verjuice or pomegranate juice.

In the case of urticaria, sitting on running water will be enough and the patient should eat light meals. Yet, if it continues and gets worse, then the cure will be bleeding, and the patient should consume cooked terminalia.

The cure for the impetigo is to pour cold water over the infected area and then rub it with rose water.

Chapter seven: Regarding warts

If there is only one or two of them, a burner medicine could be used. Yet, if there are more, then the patient should soften his bowels by consuming cuscuta. He should drink cheese water after which he should consume cooked apricot with vinegar.

Chapter eight: Regarding swellings

When the swelling is seen, the cure will be to apply goji berry mixed with rose water for a couple of days. But when it gets bigger, then it should be bandaged with a mixture of white plantago seeds powder mixed with psyllium powder, and also figs boiled with milk should be poured on the previous mixed powder and then whipped up thoroughly; and when it is ready, some amount of oil solution should be added to make it a paste that can be rubbed on the skin and be bandaged.

Chapter nine: Regarding the tumors that occur around the nails

When a tumor is found around the fingernail, then the best cure will to bleed. Yet, if there is any obstacle that prevents the patient from doing so, then he should eat lighter meals and smaller portions. The patient also should bandage his finger with a piece of cotton soaked in violet oil and dip the finger for several times in warm violet oil. If a white spot appears in that specific area, it should be wrapped with hot dough and sesame oil.

Chapter ten: Regarding the injuries around or at the edges of the nails and on the heels

If there is an opening in the injury and it is a deep one, then bandaging the injury with raw tar will be enough. Putting a small amount of tar on a piece of paper will help the healing. If the injury is not that deep, then the area can be rubbed with oil and wax.

Chapter eleven: Regarding burns

When burning happens, immediately pour hot rose oil on the area to heal and soothe the burned area, after which dusting rose petal powder over the area will be enough. Yet, when there is a burn wound, then the cure will be to use a mixture of oil, wax, and litharge which is a chemical compound made of lead monoxide, a red or yellow solid used as a pigment (here green is used instead of yellow).

Chapter twelve: Regarding poisons

When the poison is in the stomach then the cure will be vomiting with water or soft drinks and an oily substance till the stomach is totally cleaned. But if the poison goes to the intestines, then the patient should be injected with oily substances. If it spreads in the body, then it can be removed (cleaned) with mild diarrhea.

To sum up, in all kinds of poisonous bites and stings, whatever is flowing from that specific area, should be kept flowing by bandaging it with garlic, salt, and oily substances. When there is nothing left inside then it should be covered with ointment. That specific area should not be healed and should be protected.

Chapter thirteen: Regarding blood phlebotomizing (bloodletting)

Bloodletting is the best cure for the patients who have a big amount of blood in their bodies and who eat and drink a lot. The most usual vein which is suitable for bloodletting is in the elbow. As all the veins are derived from one main vein, bloodletting from one means bloodletting from the other. Yet, there is one important difference between them, which is: if the illness is in the head (upper part of the body), then the bloodletting from the upper part of the arm is faster and more beneficial than bloodletting from the basilica, though the other way around is also good. When the illness is at the bottom part of the body, then bloodletting through the basilica will be faster and better, though the other way around is also good. Whereas the middle part of the arm, which is the combination of the basilica and the upper part of the arm, includes the benefits of both positions.

Chapter fourteen: Regarding cupping

Cupping is the action of bloodletting by sucking and sometimes by force. The cupping from the legs is beneficial when the illness is at the bottom part of the body. Whereas, cupping from the back of the neck, the two sides of the neck, and the shoulders is very beneficial for the illnesses in the upper part of the body. Cupping from the hip will be very beneficial for the illnesses in the middle part of the body.

Chapter fifteen: Regarding diarrhea and enema (clyster)

Diarrhea is divided into three types. The first type is the one that is mixed with sputum. This type can be done by purging. The cure will be using *Agaricus bisporus*, Nile seeds, and cactus oil or any other ingredients with similar functions. The other type is the one mixed with yellow bile. The cure will be using the yellow terminalia and the scammonia or any other ingredients with similar functions. The third type is the one mixed with black bile. The cure will be using the black terminalia and the cuscuta, spinach and the stoechas or any other ingredients with similar functions. The enema is used to empty the abdomen and the intestines very quickly.

Chapter sixteen: Regarding vomiting

Vomiting can be of two types: the one which is caused by taking medicine, and this type is as strong as diarrhea or more effective. It is performed by using the (white) aconite and vomiting walnut. This type is very dangerous, because it could choke the person who is using it. The other way of making a person vomit is by using specific types of food or medicine that are close to the strength of those food, and by eating these the stomach and the related organs like intestine and the spleen will be purified and cleaned.

This the end of article nine.

[51B] The tenth article

This article is about fever. There are seven chapters.

Chapter one: Regarding daily fever

This type of fever happens from intensive fatigue, exposure to hot sun or intensive cold, eating spicy food, intensive anger or grief, and being exposed to some other reasons that can lead to have this type of fever which could last for 24 hours. The person who suffers this type of fever should be treated gently, and the fever can be cured by preparing juices and syrups prepared with cold water. If the person had eaten recently, then he should not eat more, and he should drink cold juices and syrups. If the patient fears that the fever might increase then he has to consume: cold soup with very little sugar and a piece of bread dipped in pomegranate juice. When the fever is gone, the patient could have a bath and can eat normal food but slightly.

Chapter two: Regarding the fever that happens every day with sputum

This type of fever generates from rotten sputum, which comes from the stomach and body veins. The cure for this will be making the patient vomit, if he is capable of vomiting and does not have any other complications, by using cooked turnip with honey and vinegar and eating a mixture of olive oil with vinegar mixed with soft, clean sesame oil and white sugar. Whenever a person mixes food and has that type of symptoms, then he should drink hot water and purify his stomach by vomiting. If the patient has a dry nature, then he has to be given rose honey in ginger water and eat soft, clean sesame oil with chickpeas water. When his nature is mild, he could eat vinegar and olive oil as it is prescribed before.

Chapter three: Regarding the fever that comes in intervals from the bile

This type of fever originates from rotten bile, which comes from the liver and body veins. The cure for this will be making the patient drink a mixture of barley water with plain vinegar and honey and eat bread dipped in pomegranate juice and verjuice, if he is capable of doing so and does not have any other complications. If the patient has a dry nature, he has to be given pear juice and soups made of spinach, squash, and almond oil.

Chapter four: Regarding the fever that comes for only one or two days

This type of fever generates from rotten black bile, which comes from the spleen and body veins. While resting, if he is capable of doing so and does not have any other complications, the patient should drink a mixture of cooked Indian black terminalia, raisin with "shanber" cucumber, and naringin and drink vinegar and honey to make the patient urinate. He also should drink celery root water and fennel and eat broilers.

Only on the day when he is having fever, he should avoid food, especially the heavy meals as the body itself will be heavy.

Chapter five: Regarding blood fever that covers the whole body

This type of fever is generated from blood disorders or excessive blood in the body. The cure for this is drinking "taberzed" sugar with pomegranate juice and eating a mixture of sour lentil with almond oil, barley water, and sour pomegranate juice. If the patient has a dry nature, he should consume jujube juice, pear, and tamarind with "taberzed" sugar and eat a mixture of squash and spinach with almond oil. When some sediment at the bottom of the flask is seen, the patient should drink cold water if his stomach is not weak enough.

Chapter six: Regarding compound fevers

When the fever types are mixed or there is some inconsistency in timing and one day is heavy and the other day is smooth, and the patient one day feels light and the other day feels heavy, this is called as compound fever. The cure and the medicine should be done according to the symptoms.

Chapter seven: Regarding daily occurring fever

When the patient is weak in body, has no strength, with weak voice, with pale face, and sunken eyes and all these symptoms are not generated from diarrhea, nose bleeding, or not being able to eat or due to any kind of concerns, then it is the striking fever; and if this fever covers the body, it is very difficult to be cured and to end it.

The end of article ten.

With the end of article ten, the book also ends with the will of God. With God's help and strength and the praise is to God alone. God bless our prophet

Muhammad and his family. We believe in God and he is the best support. There is no power or strength except in mighty God.

***

(The copier wrote to himself)

The person who copied this book is God's humble subject asking God's forgiveness and wishing for his blessing; Abdulwahab Ibn Ibrahim known as Ibn Khourooph. And may God bless all those who wish him well.

If there is any flaw in the given information, it is because of the hope of finding a remedy. May God bless whoever speaks out or approves with his silence. Success comes from Allah.

KİTAB EL-KÂNÛN EL-SAĞİR fi't-TIBB el-Reis Ebu Ali el Hüseyin İbn Sina El-Buhari

54A

KİTAB EL-KÂNÛN EL-SAĞİR fi't-TIBB el-Reis Ebu Ali el Hüseyin İbn Sina El-Buharî

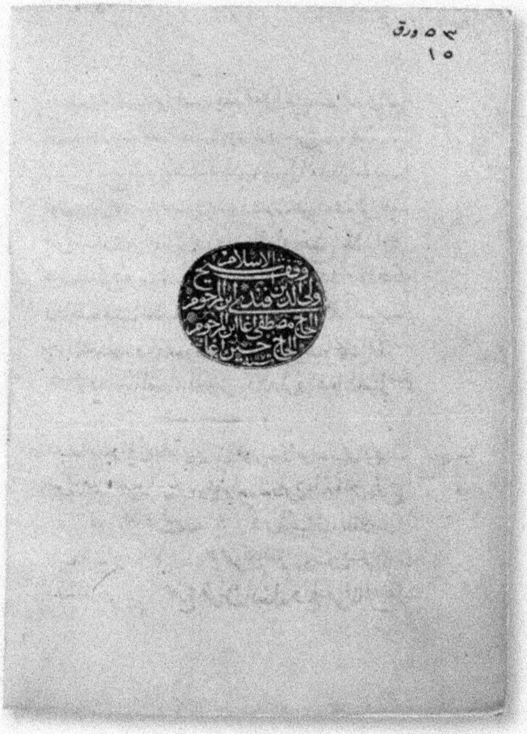

53B

www.ingramcontent.com/pod-product-compliance
Ingram Content Group UK Ltd.
Pitfield, Milton Keynes, MK11 3LW, UK
UKHW022222051026
15624UKWH00002B/301

9 783631 794760

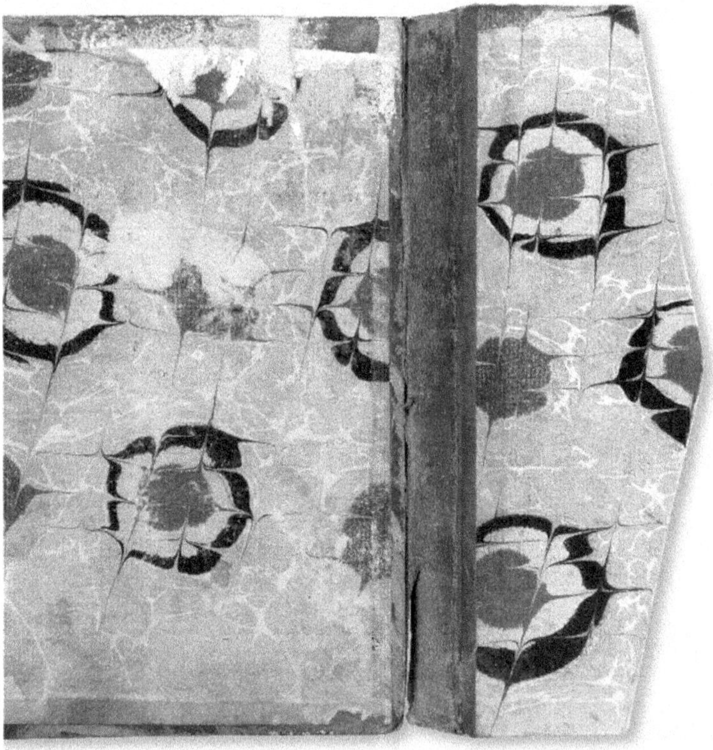

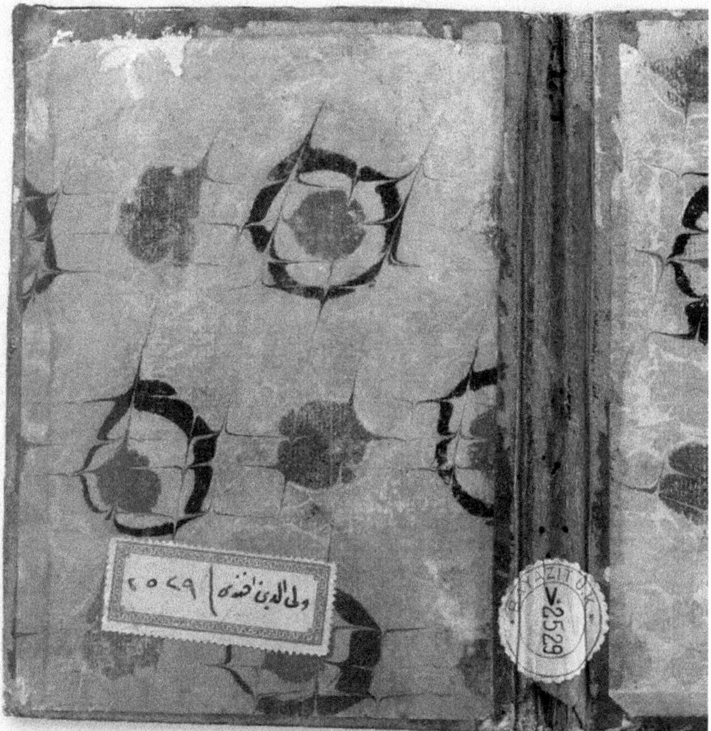

Binder cover

٢٥٢٩
٢٥٢٩
٣

KİTAB EL-KÂNÛN EL-SAĞİR fî't-TIBB / el-Reis Ebu Alî el Hüseyin İbn Sîna el-Buharî

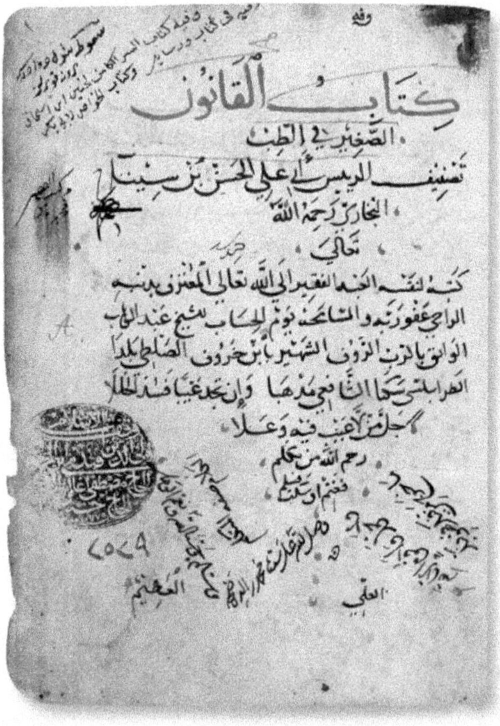
كتاب القانون
الصغير في الطب
تصنيف الرئيس أبي علي الحسن بن سينا
البخاري رحمه الله
تعالى
كتبه لنفسه العبد الفقير إلى الله تعالى المعترف بذنبه
الراجي عفو ربه والمسامحة يوم الحساب الشيخ عبد الوهاب
الواثق بالرب الرؤوف الشهير بابن خروف الصلتي بلدا
العراقي سكنا الشافعي مذهبا وإن تجد عيبا فسد الخللا
جل من لا عيب فيه وعلا

1A

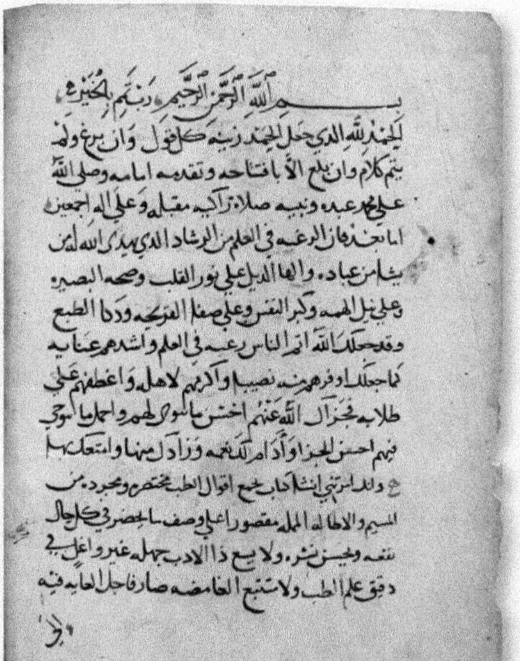
بسم الله الرحمن الرحيم رب تمم بالخير
الحمد لله الذي جعل الحمد زينة كل قول وان برع ولم
يتم كلام وان بلغ الا بافتتاحه وتقديمه امامه وصلى الله
على محمد عبده ونبيه صلاة زاكية مقبولة وعلى آله اجمعين
اما بعد فان الرغبة في العلم من الرشاد الذي يهدي الله اليه من
يشاء من عباده. وانها الدليل على نور القلب وصحة البصيرة
وعلى نبل الهمة وكبر النفس وعلى صفاء القريحة وذكاء الطبع
وقد جعلك الله اتم الناس رغبة في العلم واشدهم عناية
كما جعلك اوفرهم منه نصيبا واكرمهم لاهله واعظمهم على
طلابه فجزاك الله عنهم احسن ما يكون لهم واجمل ما يوجب
فيهم احسن الجزاء وادام لك نعمه وزادك منها واستعملك
ولذلك امرتني انشاء كتاب جمع اقوال الطب مختصرة ومجرد من
التسمية والاطالة المملة مقصورا على وصف ما يحضر في كل حال
نفعه ويحسن نشره. ولا يسع ذا الادب جهله غير واغل في
دقيق علم الطب ولا متتبع الغامضة صار فاجل الغاية فيه

1 B

الي الشرح والابانه بالالفاظ السهله الاقاويل الواضحه الدلايل
فتكلفت الذي امرتني به ثقه بعون الله عليه اذ كان من المنافع
العامه التي ياجر الله علي احلابها ويخلد كجميل الذكر بها
والله ولي التوفيق • وهذا الكتاب عشرة مقالات

المقاله الاولى

في خلق الانسان وتركيب الجسد وتقسيم الطب ومعرفه
النبض والبول وساير فصول الجسد • وهي سبعه ابواب
ا في خلق الانسان ب في تركيب الجسد من الاعضا المفرده •
ج في تركيب الجسد من الاعضا المركبه د في اقسام الطب
وحده • وذكر قوته ه في نبض العروق و في البول ز في
تعرف احوال ساير فصول الجسد

المقاله الثانيه

في معرفه قوي الاطعمه والاشربه وما بينهما وهي عشرون بابا
ا في الخبز وانواعه ب في اللحمان والبيض ج في السمك د
في الالبان ه في البقول و في اصول البقول ز في الفاكهه
اليابسه ح في الادهان ط في الرياحين ي في الطيب
يا في الفاكهه الرطبه

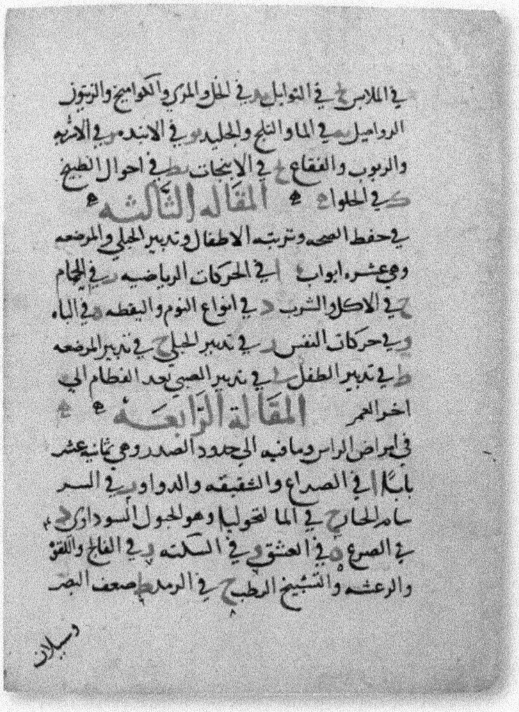
يح في الملابس يط في التوابل يو في الخل والمري والكواميخ والزيتون
يز في الرواميل يح في الما والثلج والجليد يط في الانبذه ك في الاشربه
والربوب والفقاع كا في الابنجات كب في احوال الطبيخ
كج في الحلواء

المقالة الثالثه

في حفظ الصحه وتربيه الاطفال وتدبير الحبلي والمرضعه
وهي عشره ابواب ا في الحركات الرياضيه ب في الحمام
ج في الاكل والشرب د في انواع النوم واليقظه ه في الباه
و في حركات النفس ز في تدبير الحبلي ح في تدبير المرضعه
ط في تدبير الطفل ي في تدبير الصبي بعد الفطام الي
اخر العمر

المقالة الرابعه

في امراض الراس وما فيه الي حدود الصدر وهي ثمانية عشر
بابا ا في الصداع والشقيقه والدوار ب في السر
سام الحار ج في الما لنحوليا وهو الجنون السوداوي د
في الصرع ه في العشق و في السكته ز في الفالج واللقوه
والرعشه والتشنج ح في الرمد ط ضعف البصر
ح في الرطب

وسبلان

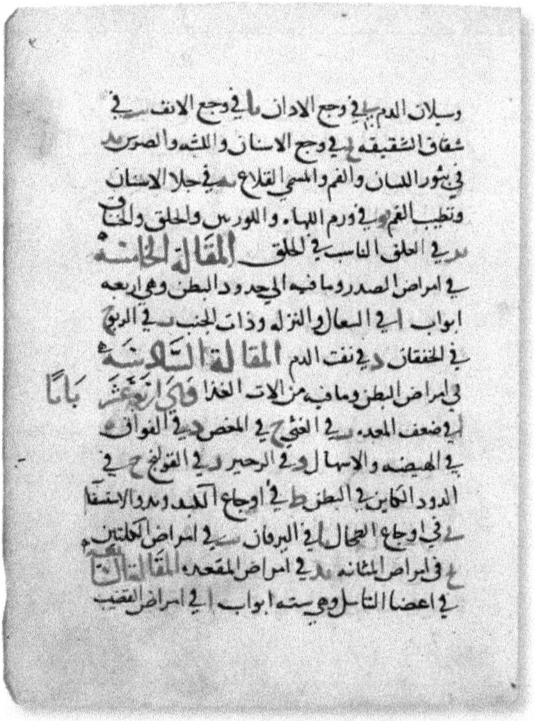

وسيلان الدم يب في وجع الاذان ما في وجع الانف س في
شقاق الشقيقه ي في وجع الاسنان واللثه والضرس
في بثور اللسان والفم والمسمى القلاع سه في جلا الاسنان
وتطيب الفم و في ورم اللهاة واللوزتين والحلق والخناق
ز في العلق الناشب في الحلق المقالة الخامسة
في امراض الصدر وما فيه الى حد و د البطن وهي اربعه
ابواب ا في السعال والنزله وذات الجنب ب في الربو
ج في الخفقان د في نفث الدم المقالة السادسة
في امراض البطن وما فيه من الات الغذا وهي اربعة عشر بابا
ا في ضعف المعده ب في الغثي ج في المغص د في الفواق
ه في الهيضه والاسهال و في الزحير ز في القولنج ح في
الدود الكاين في البطن ط في اوجاع الكبد ي في الاستسقا
يا في اوجاع الطحال يب في اليرقان يج في امراض الكليتين
يد في امراض المثانه يه في امراض المقعده المقالة السابعة
في اعضا التناسل وهي سته ابواب ا في امراض القضيب

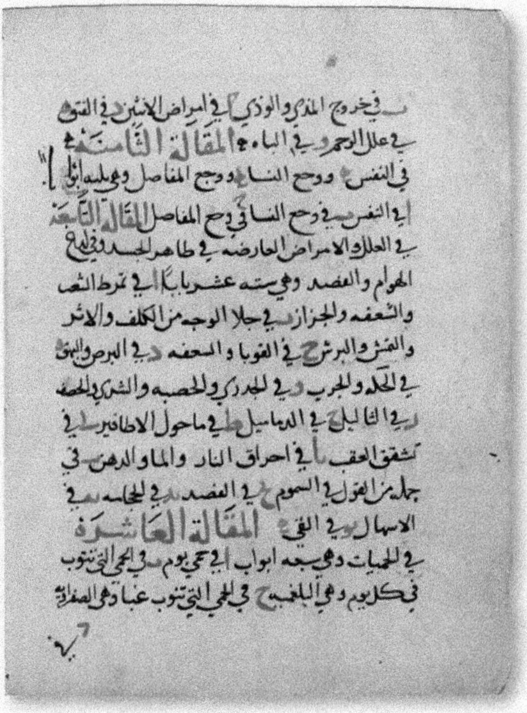

ب في خروج المذي والودي يا في امراض الانثيين د في الفتق
يه في علل الرحم و في الباه ٤٠ المقالة الثامنة في
في النفس ج ووجع النسا د وجع المفاصل وهي يليه ابواب ا
ا في النفس ب في وجع النسا ج في وجع المفاصل المقالة التاسعة
في العلل والامراض العارضة في ظاهر الجسد وفي لدغ
الهوام والعضد وهي ستة عشر بابا ا في تمرط الشعر
والشعفه والحزاز ب في جلا الوجه من الكلف والاثر
والنمش والبرش ج في القوبا والسعفه د في البرص والبهق
في الحكة والجرب و في الجدري والحصبه والشري والحصف
ز في الثاليل ح في الدماميل ط في ماحول الاظافير ي في
تشقق العقب يا في احراق النار والماء والدهن يب في
جملة من القول في السموم يج في الفصد يد في الحجامه يه في
الاسهال يو في القي المقالة العاشرة
في الحميات وهي سبعة ابواب ا في حمى يوم ب في الحمى التي تنوب
في كل يوم وهي البلغمية ج في الحمى التي تنوب غبا وهي الصفراوية

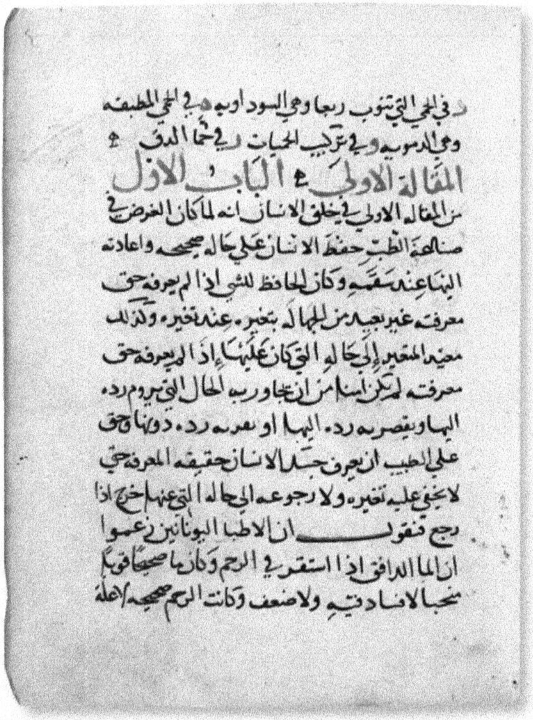
د في الحمي التي تنوب ربعا وهي السود اويه ه في الحمي المطبقه
وهي الدمويه و في تركيب الحميات ر في حما الدق
المقالة الاولي ه الباب الاول
من المقاله الاولي في خلق الانسان انه لما كان الغرض في
صناعة الطب حفظ الانسان علي حاله صحيحه واعادته
اليها عند سقمه وكان الحافظ للشي اذا لم يعرفه حق
معرفته غير بعيد من الجهاله بتغيره عند تغيره وكذلك
معيد المتغير الي حاله التي كان عليها اذا لم يعرفه حق
معرفته لم يكن امنا من ان تجاوز به الحال التي يروم رده
اليها او يقصر به رده اليها او يعرف به رده دونها حق
علي الطبيب ان يعرف جبلة الانسان حقيقه المعرفه حتي
لا يخفي عليه تغيره ولا رجوعه الي حاله التي عنها خرج اذا
رجع فنقول ان الاطبا اليونانيين زعموا
ان الما الدافق اذا استقر في الرحم وكان ما صحيحا قويا
منجبا لا فساد فيه ولا ضعف وكانت الرحم صحيحه لا عله

4A

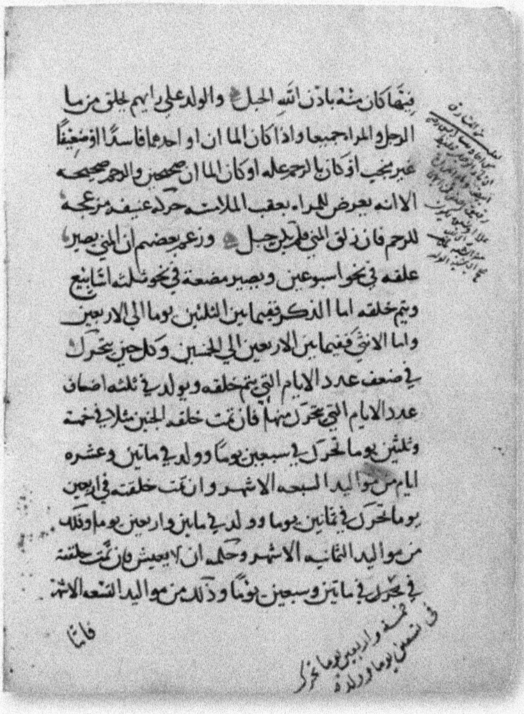
فيها كان منه باذن الله الحبل والولد على رايهم يخلق من ما
الرجل والمراة جميعا واذا كان الماان او احدهما فاسدا او ضعيفا
غير نجيب او كان بالرحم علة او كان الماان صحيحين والرحم صحيحة
الا انه يعرض للمراة بعقب الملاقاة حركة عنيفة مزعجة
للرحم فان ذلق المني فلم يكن حبل وزعم بعضهم ان المني يصير
علقة في نحو اسبوعين ويصير مضغة في نحو ثلثة اسابيع
ويتم خلقه اما الذكر فيما بين الثلثين يوما الى الاربعين
واما الانثى فيما بين الاربعين الى الخمسين وكل حين يتحرك
في ضعف عدد الايام التي يتم خلقه ويولد في ثلثة اضعاف
عدد الايام التي يتحرك منها فان تمت خلقة الجنين مثلا في خمسة
وثلثين يوما تحرك في سبعين يوما وولد في ماتين وعشرة
ايام من مواليد السبعة الاشهر وان تمت خلقته في اربعين
يوما تحرك في ثمانين يوما وولد في ماتين واربعين يوما وذلك
من مواليد الثمانية الاشهر وحكمه ان لا يعيش فان تمت خلقته
في تحرك في ماتين وسبعين يوما وذلك من مواليد التسعة الاشهر
فاما

4B

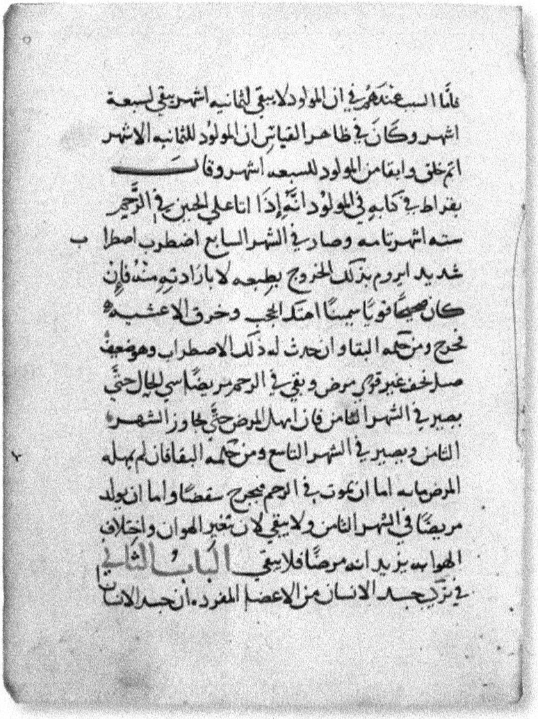

فاما السبب عندهم في ان المولود لا يبقى لثمانية اشهر ويبقى لسبعة
اشهر وكان في ظاهر القياس ان المولود للثمانية الاشهر
اتم خلق وابقا من المولود للسبعة اشهر وقال
بقراط في كتابه في المولود انه اذا اتا على الجنين في الرحم
سته اشهر تامه وصار في الشهر السابع اضطرب اضطرا ب
شديد ايروم بذلك الخروج بطبعه لا بارادته منه فان
كان صحيحا قويا سمينا اهتك الحجب وخرق الاغشيه
فخرج ومن جمله البقا وان حدث له ذلك الاضطراب وهو ضعيف
مسلخف غير قوي مرض وبقي في الرحم مريضا سي الحال حتى
يصير في الشهر الثامن فان اتهل المرض حتى يجاوز الشهر
الثامن ويصير في الشهر التاسع ومن جمله البقا فان لم يهله
المرض ما به اما ان يموت في الرحم فيخرج سقطا واما ان يولد
مريضا في الشهر الثامن ولا يبقى لان تغير الهوا وان اختلاف
الهوا به يزيد انه مرضا فلا يبقى الباب الثاني
في تركيب جسد الانسان من الاعضا المفرد. ان جسد الانسا

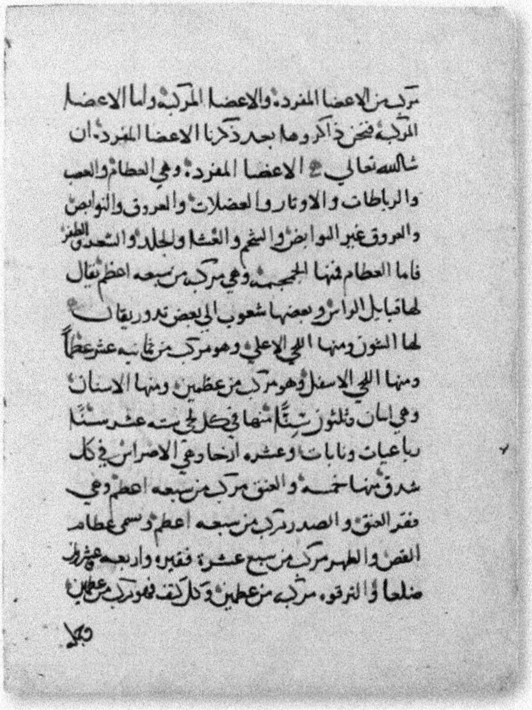

مركب من الاعضا المفرده والاعضا المركبه واما الاعضا
المركبه فنحن ذاكروها بعد ذكرنا الاعضا المفرده ان
شا الله تعالي الاعضا المفرده وهي العظام والعصب
والرباطات والاوتار والعضلات والعروق والنوابض
والعروق غير النوابض والشحم والغشا والجلد والشعر والظفر
فاما العظام فمنها الجمجمه وهي مركبه من سبعه اعظم يقال
لها قبايل الراس وبعضها شعوب الي بعض بدرور يقال
لها الشون ومنها اللحي الاعلي وهو مركب من ثمانيه عشر عظما
ومنها اللحي الاسفل وهو مركب من عظمين ومنها الاسنان
وهي اثنان وثلثون سنا منها في كل لحي سته عشر سنا
رباعيات وانيابات وعشره ارحا وهي الاضراس في كل
شدق منها خمسه والعنق مركب من سبعه اعظم وهي
فقر العنق والصدر مركب من سبعه اعظم وتسمي عظام
القص والظهر مركب من سبع عشره فقيره واربعه عشر
ضلعا والترقوه مركبه من عظمين وكل كتف فهو مركب من عظمين
وكل

وجملة كل يد مركبة من عضد وزند اسفل وثمانية اعظم يقال
لجملتها الرسغ واربعة اعظم يقال لجملتها الكف وخمسة اصابع
مركبة من خمسة عشر عظمًا والوركان عظمان وكل ساق
مركبة من عظمين هما الزندان وكل قدم مركبة من كعب وعقب
وعظم يسمى العظم الزورقي واربعة اعظم من رسغ القدم وخمسة
اعظم من مشط القدم وخمس اصابع مركبة من ثمانية وعشرين
عظمًا فجميع عظام الجسد ٢٤٨ عظمًا ومنفعتها
في بدن الحيوان نوعان احدهما شد بنية الجسد
والمنفعة الاخرى حفظه وبقاؤه وكذلك جعل الله جل اسمه
بعض العظام قواعد واساسًا للاعضا كالعصعص وعظم
العجز وفقار الظهر وجعل بعضها جنة ووقاية للاعضا وذلك
بمنزلة قحف الراس الذي جعل فيه الدماغ وبمنزلة عظام القص
التي جعلت جنة للقلب والرية وبمنزلة الضلوع التي جعلت
جنة للاحشا واما العصب فان منفعته في بدن الحيوان
افادة حركة الحس والحركة والعصب نوعان احدهما

ينبت من الدماغ وهي سبعه ازواج يكون لها حس الحواس
الخمس وحس بعض الاعضا وحركته والنوع الاخر ينبت
من النخاع وهي احدو ثلثون زوجًا وفرد لا زوج له وبهذا
النوع من العصب يكون حس الاعضا التي دون الرقبه وحركتها
واما العضلات فهي لحم الجسد وتركيبها من اللحم المحض الخالص
والعصب والعروق ولها في الجسد منفعتان احدهما
تحريك الاوصال بمعاونه الاوتار والاخري ان يكسوا العظام
لها ايضا منفعه اخري وهي ان تحقن الحراره الغريزيه في
الجسد ليلا يتحلل فيبرد الجسد واما العروق النوابض
فمنشاها من القلب وجسمها عصبي متضاعف وليس
لها حس ولا حركه في نفسها وفي تجويفها روح كثيره ودم
قليل ومنفعتها ان تفيد الاعضا قوه الحيوه التي تفيدها
واما العروق غير النوابض فمنشاها من الكبد وجسمها عصبي
غير مضاعف وليس لها حس ولا حركه وهي جداول الكبد
وفيها دم كثير وروح قليله ومنفعتها ان تسقي الاعضا الدم

الذي

الذي تتحلله من الكبد واما السمين فمنه شحم الترب والمصارين
ومنفعته ان تدفي الاحشا وتزيد في حرزها وحصانتها
ومنه شحم الكلي ومنفعته ان يدفي الكليتين ويصونها عن
الافات ، واما العصب فانه جسم عصبي صلب دقيق عديم
الحركة وله حس قليل ومنفعته ان يقي الاعضا ويصونها واما
الجلد فانه جسم عصبي وله كثير ومنشاه من عصب الدماغ
ومنفعته ستر اللحم وصيانته وفيه ثقب كثيرة وهي مخارج
الشعر والعروق والبخار اللطيف وقد يتنفس الجسد
من هذه الخروق ، واما الشعر فانه انواع منه ما يزين
الجسد ويقي منبته منه شعر الراس فانه يقي جلد الراس
ويزين جملة الجسد ومنه ما يزين جملة البدن وينفع بعض
الاعضا دون بعض مثل شعر الحاجبين وهدب العينين
فانهما يمنعان الافات عن البصر ويزيدان في قوته ويزينان
جملة البدن ومنه ما يجمع المنفعة فقط دون الزينة مثل

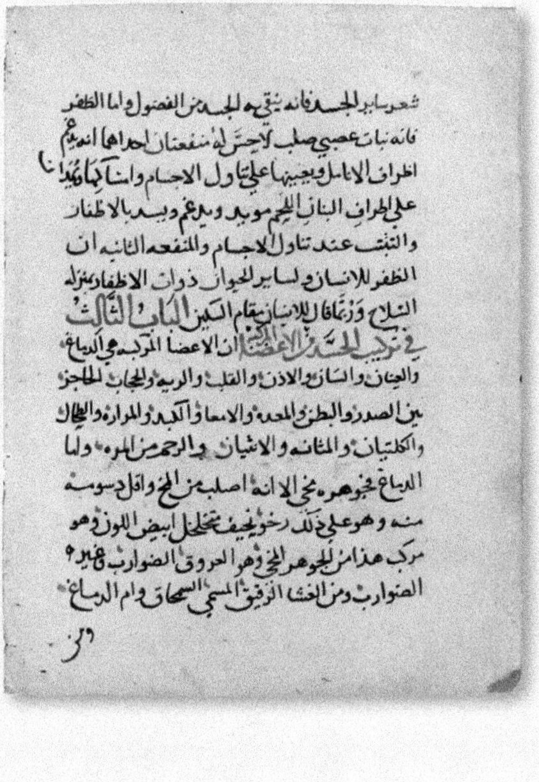
شعر ساير الجسد فانه ينقي به الجسد من الفضول واما الظفر
فانه نبات عصبي صلب لا حس له منفعتان احداهما انه يدعم
اطراف الانامل ويعينها علي تناول الاجسام وامساكها ويمدها
علي اطراف البنان اللحم موبد ويدعم ويسند بالاظفار
والتثبت عند تناول الاجسام والمنفعه الثانيه ان
الظفر للانسان ولساير الحيوان ذوات الاظفار بمنزله
السلاح وربما قام للانسان مقام السكين الباب الثالث
في تركيب الجسد من الاعضاء الكثيره ان الاعضا المركبه هي الدماغ
والعينان واللسان والاذن والقلب والريه والحجاب الحاجز
بين الصدر والبطن والمعده والامعا والكبد والمراره والطحال
والكليتان والمثانه والانثيان والرحم من المره ولما
الدماغ فجوهره مخي الا انه اصلب من المخ واقل دسومه
منه وهو علي ذلك رخو خفيف متخلخل ابيض اللون وهو
مركب هذا من الجوهر المخي وهي العروق الضوارب وغير
الضوارب ومن الغشا الرقيق المسمي السحاق وام الدماغ
ومن

٨

ومن الغشا الصلب الذي يلي القحف والدماغ منشا العصب
ومنشا النخاع وهيه الدماغ مثلثه الا انها ليست بصحيحه
التثليث ولا بينه الزوايا وكان قاعده المثلثه تلي مقدم
الراس ويلتقي ساقيها علي موخر الراس وبالدماغ يكون الحس
بتوسط العصب اللين والحركه بتوسط العصب الصلب
وله بطون تحوي الروح النفسانيه فبطنه المقدم يكون
التخيل ويكون الاتشاذ وات الصور وبوسطه يكون الفكر
في الاشيا وبموخره يكون حفظ الاشيا وادراكها
والدماغ اول عضو علي راي ابقراط فاما العينان فكل
واحد منهما مركبه من سبع طبقات وثلثه رطوبات
فالطبقه الاولي مما يلي الهوا تسمى الملتحمه وهي بياض العين
وبعد هذه الطبقه القرنيه الطبقه العنبيه ولونها
تختلف في الابدان فمره تكون سودا ومره تكون زرقا
ومره شهلا وبعدها الرطوبه البيضيه وهي رطوبه
شبيهه ببياض البيض وبعد هذه الرطوبه الطبقه

العنكبوتيه وهي طبقه شبيهه بنسج العنكبوت في رقتها
وبعد هذه الطبقه الرطوبه الجليديه وهي رطوبه صافيه
نيره شبيهه بالجليد مستديره غير صحيحه الاستداره
وبه الرطوبه تكون البصر وبعدها الرطوبه الزجاجيه
وهي شبيهه بالزجاج الذايب في الاتون وبعدها الطبقه
الشبكيه وهي تشبه الشبكه وبعدها الطبقه المشيميه
وهي تشبه المشيمه لانها ذات عروق كثيره وبعدها الطبقه
الصلبه وهي تلي عظم العين فاما اللسان فانه مركب من لحم
رخيف ابيض ومن عروق وشاريانات ومن عصب كثير
حساس ومن عضلات مطبقه باصله ومن غشا متصل
بغشا المري والمعده ومنفعته الكلام وقلب الطعام والمعونه
على بلوغ ما يبلغ واما الاذن فانها مركبه من غضروف ولحم
محض وعصب حساس والسمع تكون بالسماخ واما الاذن
فانها تقبل الصوت وتجمعه ليدخل شيا فشيا في السماخ
واما القلب فانه جسم مخروط الهيه قاعدته في وسط
الصدر

٩

الصدر وطرفه مايل الى ذات اليسار ولونه احمر بهرماني
وهو مركب من هذا اللحم وهو جوهر ابيض شبيه بالليف
ومن غشا صلب يسمى الشغاف وله بطنان في احدهما وهو
الايمن دم كثير وروح قليله وفي الاخر وهو الايسر روح كثيره
ودم قليل وكل واحد من البطنين ينفذ الى الاخر ومن بطنه
تنبت العروق والنوابض ومن البطن الايمن والقلب مجاري
حركتهما من القلب الى الريه دم الغذا ومن الريه الى القلب
وهو النفس والقلب ينبوع الحراره الغريزيه والروح الحيوانيه
وهو اول عضو خلق على راي ارسطاطاليس وجالينوس
واما الريه فانها مركبه من لحم سخيف على لون الورد ومن
قصبه الريه ومن شعب قصبه الريه ومن عروق غير
ضاربه تاتيهما من القلب بالدم والحراره الغريزيه وليس
للريه حس البته واما غشاوها فله حس ضعيف وقصبه
الريه عضروفيه الجوهر ومنفعه الريه الترويح عن
الحراره الغريزيه التي في القلب وفي صيانه القلب

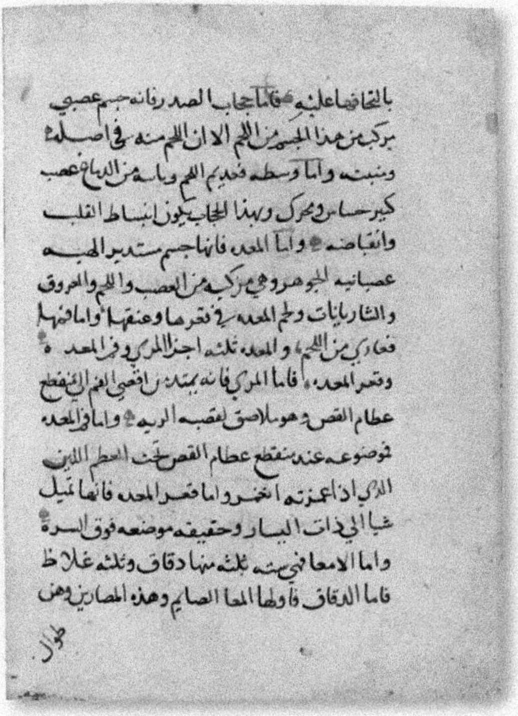
بالتحافها عليه فاما حجاب الصدر فانه جسم عصبي
مركب من هذا الجسم من اللحم الا ان اللحم منه في اصله
ومنبته واما وسطه فعديم اللحم وبانه من الدماغ عصب
كبير حساس ومحرك وبهذا الحجاب يكون انبساط القلب
وانقباضه واما المعده فانها جسم مستدير الهيئه
عصبانيه الجوهر وهي مركبه من العصب واللحم والعروق
والشاريانات ولحم المعده في قعرها وعنقها واما فمها
فعاري من اللحم والمعده ثلثه اجزا المري وفم المعده
وقعر المعده فاما المري فانه يبتدي من اقصي الفم الي منقطع
عظام القص وهو ملاصق لقصبه الريه واما فم المعده
فموضوعه عند منقطع عظام القص تحت العظم اللين
الذي اذا غمزته انغمز واما قعر المعده فانها تميل
شيا الي ذات اليسار وحقيقه موضعه فوق السره
واما الامعا فهي سته ثلثه منها دقاق وثلثه غلاظ
فاما الدقاق فاولها المعا الصايم وهذه المصارين وهي
طوال

طوال جدا دقاق واقل المعا الغلاظ المسمى الاعور وهو متصل
باخر المصارين وبعده المعا المعروف بالقولون وبعده المعا
المعروف بالمستقيم وطرفه متصل بالدبر وجسم الامعا عصبي
مضاعف وله حس بالامعا مركب من هذا الجسم ومن اللحم
والعروق والشاريانات وفعل الامعا دفع ثفل الطعام
بين من الجسد واما الكبد موضعها في الجانب الايمن
واعلاها مماس لحجاب الصدر وظهرها ملاصق لضلوع الخلف
وبطنها ملاصق لضلوع الخلف وبطنها ملاصق المعده واسفلها
ينتهي الى الخاصره ولونها احمر قان ولحمها شبيه بالدم الجا مد
وهي منبت العروق غير الضوارب ومستقر القوه الطبيعيه
وهي مركب من اللحم الذي وصفنا ومن العروق والشاريانا ت
والغشا التي تسترها وليس للكبد في نفسها حس فاما الغشا وما
فله حس قوي ومنفعه الكبد توليد الدم لغذا الجسد
والمراره ملاصقه الكبد وهي وعا المره الصفرا ومنفعتها
جذب المره الصفرا من الكبد واما الطحال فموضوع في

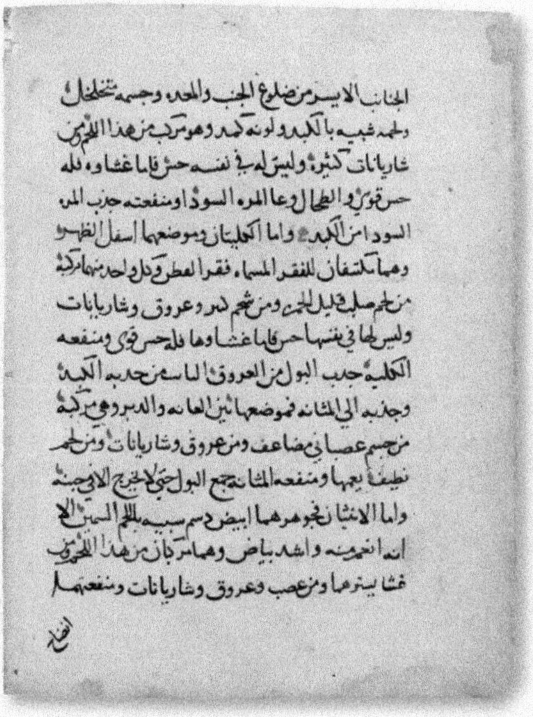

الجانب الايسر من ضلوع الجنب والمعده وجسمه متخلخل
ولحمه شبيه بالكبد ولونه كمد وهو مركب من هذا اللحم ومن
شاريانات كثيرة وليس له في نفسه حس فاما غشاوه فله
حس قوي والطحال وعا المره السودا ومنفعته جذب المره
السودا من الكبد واما الكليتان وموضعهما اسفل الظهر
وهما ملتصقان للفقرا المسماه فقرا القطن وكل واحد منهما مركبة
من لحم صلب قليل الحمره ومن شحم كثير وعروق وشاريانات
وليس لها في نفسها حس فاما غشاوها فله حس قوي ومنفعه
الكلية جذب البول من العروق النابتة من حدبة الكبد
وجذبه الي المثانه فموضعها بين العانه والدبر وهي مركبة
من جسم عصباني مضاعف ومن عروق وشاريانات ومن لحم
لطيف يعمها ومنفعه المثانه جمع البول حتى لا يخرج الا في حينه
واما الانثيان فجوهرهما ابيض دسم شبيه باللحم السمين الا
انه انعم منه واشد بياضا وهما مركبان من هذا اللحم ومن
غشا يسترهما ومن عصب وعروق وشاريانات ومنفعتهما

انضاج

انضاج المني واعداده لوقت خروجه ۞ واما القضيب فمركب
من عصب كثير وعروق وشاريانات كثيره ومن لحم قليل وفي
عضلات مطيفه باصله وهو كثير الحس جدا ومنفعته مشهوره
واما الرحم وهي عصبانيه وهي موضوعه فيما بين المثانه والمعا
المستقيم والسره ولها عنق يسمى الى الفرج وفي اصل عنقها
الانثيان فاما بها عصب كثير حاس وعروق ضوارب
وغير ضوارب ومنفعتها قبول الحبل ۞ واما اوصال الجسد
في الراس والعنق والكتفان والعضدان والساعدان
والكفان والظهر مع الصدر والبطن والعجز والفخذان
والساقان والقدمان فاما اخلاط الجسد فنحن ذاكروها
في الباب التاسع ان شا الله تعالى ۞ الباب الرابع
في قسمه الطب وتفسير اقسامه وذكر فقره ان صناعة
الطب قسمان احدهما العلم والاخر العمل فاما العلم فهو
معرفه الاشيا الطبيعيه والاشيا غير الطبيعيه والاشيا
غير الطبيعيه والاشيا الخارجه عن الطبيعه فالاشيا

الطبيعه والاشيا الخارجه احد عشر شيا علم واركان
وهي النار والهوي والما والارض فقوه النار حاره يابسه
وقوه الهوي حار رطب وقوه الما بارد رطب وقوه الارض
بارده يابسه ع والاخلاط اربعه الدم ع وهو حار
رطب المره الصفرا وهي حاره يابسه المره السودا
وهي بارده يابسه البلغم وهو بارد رطب والثالث
وهو تسعه اربعة منها مفرده وهي الحراره والبروده
والرطوبه واليبوسه وامزجه مركبه وهي الحراره
مع اليبوسة والحرارة مع الرطوبه والبروده مع اليبوسه
والبروده مع الرطوبه ومزاج تاسع وهو المعتدل والرابع
وهي الاعضا وقد وصفنا امرها في البابين الثاني والثالث
والخامس القوي وذلك ان لكل عضو من الاعضا المفرده
قوه مثل ان اللحم حار رطب والعظم بارد يابس والعصب
بارد رطب ولكل عضو مركب ايضا قوه خاصيه مثل ان
الدماغ بارد رطب ع والقلب حار يابس والكبد حار

رطب

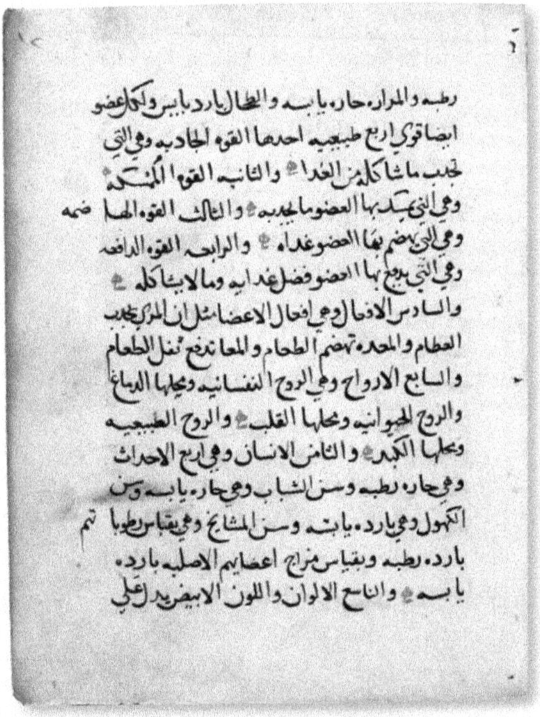

رطبه والمراره حاره يابسه والطحال بارد يابس ولكل عضو
ايضا قوى اربع طبيعيه احدها القوه الجاذبه وهي التي
تجذب ما شاكله من الغذا والثانيه القوه الممسكه
وهي التي يمسك بها العضو ما يجذبه والثالث القوه الهاضمه ضمه
وهي التي يهضم بها العضو غذاه والرابعه القوه الدافعه
وهي التي يدفع بها العضو فضل غذايه وما لا يشاكله
والسادس الافعال وهي افعال الاعضا مثل ان المرى يجذب
الطعام والمعده تهضم الطعام والمعا تدفع ثقل الطعام
والسابع الارواح وهي الروح النفسانيه ومحلها الدماغ
والروح الحيوانيه ومحلها القلب والروح الطبيعيه
ومحلها الكبد والثامن الاسنان وهي اربع الاحداث
وهي حاره رطبه وسن الشباب وهي حاره يابسه وسن
الكهول وهي بارده يابسه وسن المشايخ وهي بقياس رطوبا تهم
بارده رطبه وبقياس مزاج اعضايهم الاصليه بارده
يابسه والتاسع الالوان واللون الابيض يدل على

٢

البلغم والاحمر يدل على الدم والاصفر يدل على المره الصفرا
والاسود يدل على المره السودا ❊ والعاشر السحه وهي حال
الجسد في السمن والهزل والسمن ان كان من الشحم فهو
دليل البرد والرطوبه وان كان من اللحم فهو دليل الحر والرطوبه
وان كان مع اليباس فهو دليل البرد واليبوسه ❊ والحادي
عشر معرفه الفرق بين الذكر والانثي ❊ فالذكور في اكثر
الامر حار والانثي في اكثر الامر بارد ❊ واما الاشيا الطبيعيه
فمعانيها تسعه اشيا الهوا المحيط بالاجسام والحركه ❊
والسكون والحمام والاطعمه والاشربه والنوم واليقظه
وحركات النفس مثل السرور والغم والغضب والرضا
والاشيا الخارجه عن الطبيعه فمعانيها ثلثه اشيا
معرفه الامراض ومعرفه اسباب الامراض ومعرفه
دلايل الامراض واما علم الطب فاينقسم الي جزين احدهما
حمل الاصحا على صحتهم والاخر علاج المرض واما حد الطب
فان الطب لحد ثانه العلم بالامور التي تحفظ الصحه او تجلبها

وبالامور

وبالامور التي تحفظ الامراض او تجلبها وبالامور التي تحفظ
وتجلب الاحوال التي ليست منسوبة الى الصحة ولا الى المرض
واما فرق الطب فانها ثلثه احدهما اصحاب الراي والقيا[س]
والثاني اصحاب التجارب العاريه من القياس والنظر واصحا[ب]
الحيل وهي فرقه تابعه تتبع بالحيل والمخاريق

الباب الخامس

في جملة موجزة من تعرف نبض العروق ان العروق الضوارب
كلها تنبض نبضا واحدا مناسبا لنبض القلب ولذلك
يجوز الاستدلال بنبض احدها على نبض جماعتها وعلى نبض
القلب وابين العروق النوابض حركة العروق التي في
المعصمين والعروق التي في الصدغين والعروق التي
في رسغي القدمين فاما العروق التي في باطن الجسد فابينها
حركة العروق الذي تنبض تحت الثدو. اليسرى وهو اول
عرق نابض يخرج من القلب والعروق الضارب المستبطن
لعظام الصلب فان هذا العرق يظهر نبضه لمن وضع يده

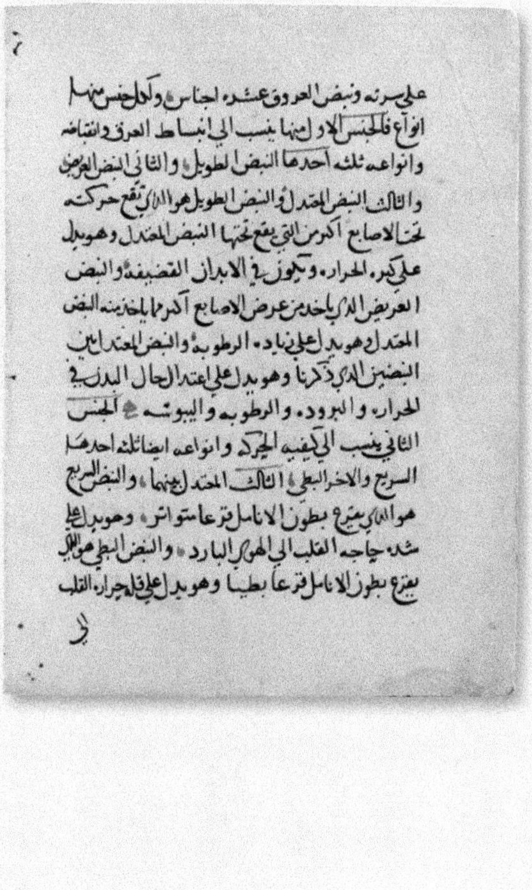
علي سرته ونبض العروق عشره اجناس ولكل جنس منها
انواع فالجنس الاول منها ينسب الي انبساط العرق وانقباضه
وانواعه ثلثه احدها النبض الطويل والثاني النبض العريض
والثالث النبض المعتدل والنبض الطويل هو الذي تقع حركته
تحت الاصابع اكثر من التي يقع تحتها النبض المعتدل وهو يدل
علي كثره الحراره ويكون في الابدان القضيفه والنبض
العريض الذي ياخذ من عرض الاصابع اكثر مما ياخذه النبض
المعتدل وهو يدل علي زياده الرطوبه والنبض المعتدل بين
النبضين الذين ذكرنا وهو يدل علي اعتدال حال البدن في
الحراره والبروده والرطوبه واليبوسه الجنس
الثاني ينسب الي كيفيه الحركه وانواعه ايضا ثلثه احدها
السريع والاخر البطي الثالث المعتدل بينهما والنبض السريع
هو الذي يقرع بطون الانامل قرعا متواترا وهو يدل علي
شده حاجه القلب الي الهوي البارد والنبض البطي هو الذي
يقرع بطون الانامل قرعا بطيا وهو يدل علي قله حراره القلب

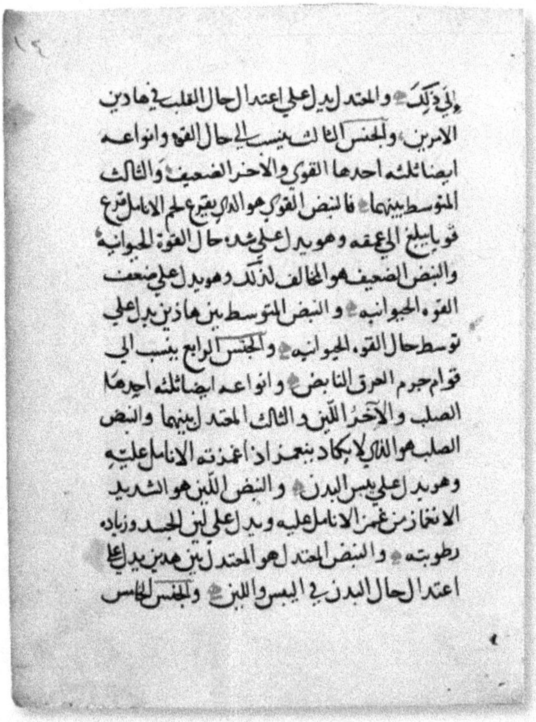

الي ذلك والمعتدل يدل علي اعتدال حال القلب في هاذين
الامرين والجنس الثالث ينسب الي حال القوه وانواعه
ايضا ثلثه احدها القوي والاخر الضعيف والثالث
المتوسط بينهما فالنبض القوي هو الذي يقرع لحم الانامل قرع
قويا يبلغ الي عمقه وهو يدل علي شده حال القوة الحيوانيه
والنبض الضعيف هو المخالف لذلك وهو يدل علي ضعف
القوه الحيوانيه والنبض المتوسط بين هاذين يدل علي
توسط حال القوه الحيوانيه والجنس الرابع ينسب الي
قوام جرم العرق النابض وانواعه ايضا ثلثه احدها
الصلب والاخر اللين والثالث المعتدل بينهما والنبض
الصلب هو الذي لا يكاد ينغمز اذا غمزته الانامل عليه
وهو يدل علي يبس البدن والنبض اللين هو الشديد
الانغماز من غمز الانامل عليه ويدل علي لين الجسد وزياده
رطوبته والنبض المعتدل هو المعتدل بين هذين يدل علي
اعتدال حال البدن في اليبس واللين والجنس الخامس

هو المنسوب الي وقت فتور الحركة وهو ايضا ثلثه انواع احدها
المتواتر وهو الذي يقرع الانامل قرعا متواترا وهو يدل علي
ضعف القوه وذلك اذا كان مع التواتر عظم ومرة يدل
علي شيء من الطبيعة البدن وذلك اذا كان مع التواتر عظم
والاخر المتفاوت وهو الذي يقرع الانامل قرعا بطيا
وهو يدل علي برد البدن وذلك اذا كان مع التفاوت عظم
ومرة يدل علي اخلال القوه وذلك اذا كان مع التفاوت صغر
والثالث المعتدل وهو يدل علي اعتدال حال البدن فيما ذكرنا
والجنس السادس المنسوب الي الانتظام وهو الجنس الحافظ
لنظام حركته علي نسبة واحده وهو يدل علي حسن حال
البدن والجنس السابع وهو المنسوب الي الاختلاف وهو
النبض الذي لا يحفظ نامه وهو يدل علي تغير حال البدن
والجنس الثامن هو المنسوب الي وزن الحركة وهو ان يكون زمان
حركة النبض موازيا لزمان سكونه وذلك يدل علي اعتدال
الحال في الانقباض والانبساط والجنس التاسع هو

المنسوب

المنسوب الي كيفيه حراره جسم العرق وبروديه وانواعه
ثلثه احدها الحار وهو ان يكون جسم العرق ايضا وذلك
يدل علي حراره في تجويفه من والروح والثاني البارد
وهو ان يكون جسم العرق النابض بارد وذلك يدل علي
تجويف العرق من الدم والروح والثالث المعتدل وهو
يدل علي اعتدال حال الروح في الحراره والبروده والجنس
العاشر هو المنسوب الي مقدار ما في تجويف العرق النابض
وانواعه ثلثه الممتلي وهو يدل علي كثره الدم والروح والثاني
الخالي وهو يدل علي اعتدال مقدارها

الباب السابع

في جمله موجزه في تعرف البول يدل علي احد امرين اما علله
عامه للبدن كله بمنزله الحمي وساير اصناف سوء المزاج
واما علله حاصله في مجاري البول وهي الكليتان والمثانه
ومجري القضيب من الرجل ومجري الفرج من المراه والبول
المحمود المعتدل والبول قسمان احدهما الما والثاني
الثفل المتميز عن الماء والما قسمان احدهما القوام والاخر

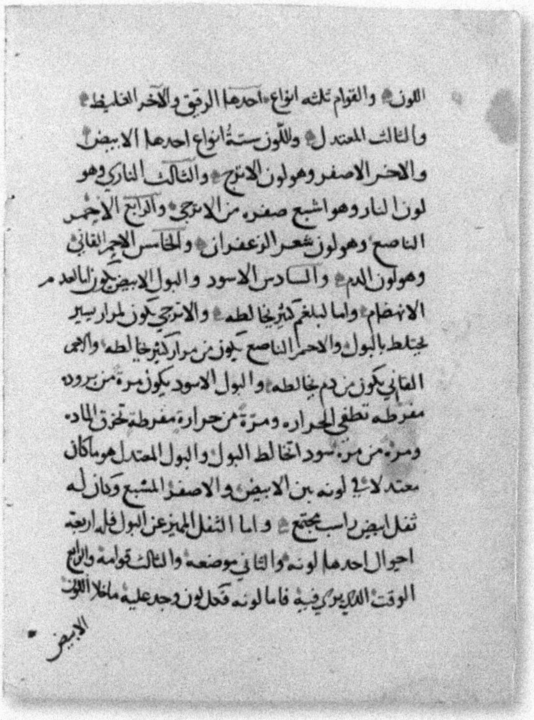

اللون • والقوام ثلثه انواع • احدها الرقيق والاخر الغليظ •
والثالث المعتدل • وللون ستة انواع احدها الابيض
والاخر الاصفر وهو لون الاترج • والثالث الناري وهو
لون النار وهو اشبع صفرة من الاترجي • والرابع الاحمر
الناصع وهو لون شعر الزعفران • والخامس الاحمر القاني
وهو لون الدم • والسادس الاسود والبول الابيض يكون اما لعدم
الانهضام • واما لبلغم كثير يخالطه • والاترجي يكون لمرار يسير
يختلط بالبول • والاحمر الناصع يكون من مرار كثير يخالطه • والاحمر
القاني يكون من دم يخالطه • والبول الاسود يكون مرة من برودة
مفرطة تطفي الحرارة ومرة من حرارة مفرطة تحرق المادة
ومرة من مرة سوداء تخالط البول • والبول المعتدل هو ما كان
معتدلا في لونه بين الابيض والاصفر المشبع وكان له
ثفل ابيض راسب مجتمع • واما الثفل المميز عن البول فله اربعة
احوال احدها لونه • والثاني موضعه • والثالث قوامه • والرابع
الوقت الذي يرى فيه • فاما لونه فكل لون وجد عليه ما خلا اللون
الابيض

١٦

الابيض فانه موذن بفساد حال البدن وامام وضعه فمحل موضع
يرى فيه القاروره ما خلا اسفلها فهو ردي واما قوامه فان
كان غليظا جدا غير منتشر اذا حرك او كان رقيقا منتشر
فانه ردي واما الوقت الذي يرى فينبغي ان يكون موجودا في
بول الاصحاء في كل وقت واما في ابوال المرضى فينبغي ان يكون
وجوده في اول المرض او بعد ذلك بايام يسيره فانه اذا
ظهر ذلك دل على حسن حال المريض وعلى سرعه نضج مرضه
واذا تاخر ظهوره دل على تاخر النضج لصعوبه المرض

الباب التاسع في احوال ما ينتقص من الجسد

انه ينبغي ان ينتقص فضول الجسد كل يوم عن اخرها فانه يكون
دوام الصحه باذن الله فاول الفضول البارزه عن الجسد
ثفل الطعام وينبغي ان يعني حافظ صحه جسده باستفراغه
كل يوم عن اخره فان به تكون سلامه المعده والامعا كلها
والجانب المقعر من الكبد وهذا الثفل ينبغي ان يكون نازلا
في وقت عادته وان يكون معتدلا في قوامه بين الرقيق والصلب

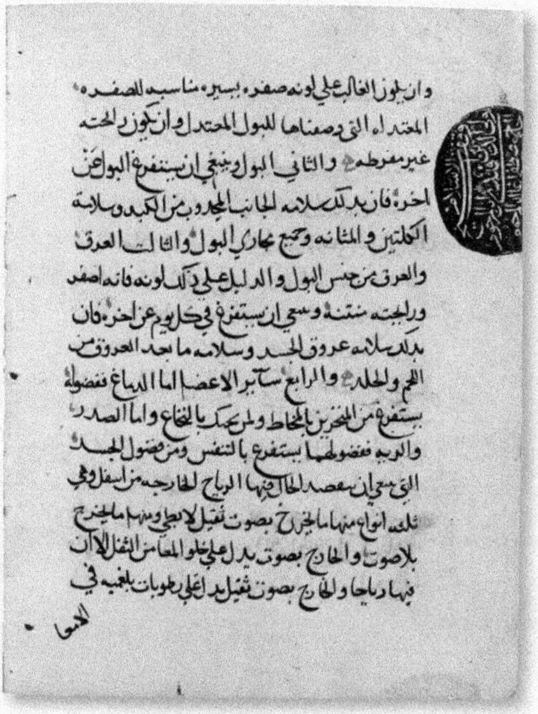

وان يكون الغالب على لونه صفره يسيره مناسبه للصفره
المعتداه التي وصفناها للبول المعتدل وان يكون رائحته
غير مفرطه ۞ والثاني البول وينبغي ان يستفرغ البول عن
اخره فان بذلك سلامه للجانب المحدب من الكبد وسلامة
الكليتين والمثانه وجميع مجاري البول ۞ والثالث العرق
والعرق من جنس البول والدليل على ذلك لونه فانه اصفر
ورائحته منتنه وينبغي ان يستفرغ في كل يوم عن اخره فان
بذلك سلامه عروق الجسد وسلامه ما بعد العروق من
اللحم والجلد ۞ والرابع سائر الاعضا اما الدماغ ففضوله
يستفرغ من المنخرين بالمخاط ومن الحنك بالنخاع واما الصدر
والريه ففضولهما يستفرغ بالتنفس ومن فضول الجسد
التي ينبغي ان يقصد الحال فيها الرياح الخارجه من اسفل وهي
ثلثه انواع منها ما يخرج بصوت ثقيل لا يبطي ومنها ما يخرج
بلا صوت والخارج بصوت يدل على خلو المعا من الثفل الا ان
فيها رياحا والخارج بصوت ثقيل يدل على رطوبات بلغميه في
الامعا

16B

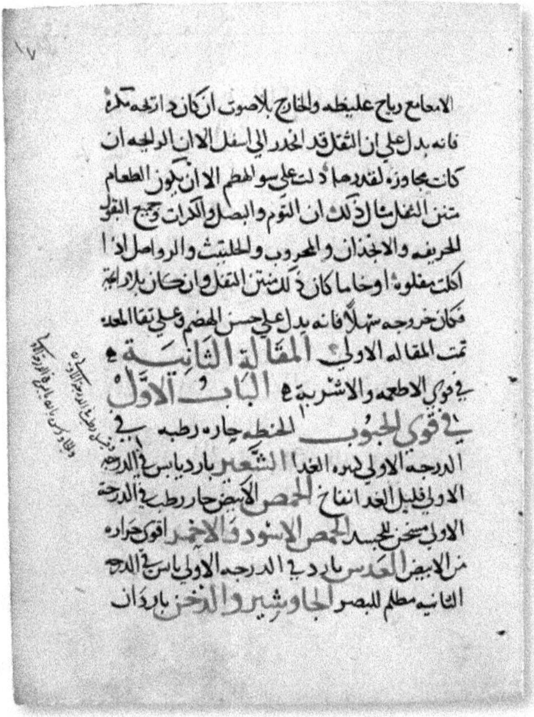
١٧

الامعاء رياح غليظه والخارج بلا صوت ان كان ذا رائحه منكره
فانه يدل على ان الثقل قد انحدر الى اسفل الا ان الوجه ان
كانت مجاوزه لقدرها دلت على سو الهضم الا ان يكون الطعام
منتن الثقل مثال ذلك ان الثوم والبصل والكراث وجميع البقول
الحريفه والانجذان والمحروب والحلتيث والرواصل اذا
اكلت مقلوه او خاما كان ذلك منتن الثقل وان كان بلا رائحه
فكان خروجه سهلا فانه يدل على حسن الهضم وعلى نقا المعده
تمت المقاله الاولى المقاله الثانيه
في قوى الاطعمه والاشربه الباب الاول
في قوى الحبوب الحنطه حاره رطبه في
الدرجه الاولى كثيره الغذا الشعير بارد يابس في الدرجه
الاولى قليل الغذا نفاخ الحمص الابيض حار رطب في الدرجه
الاولى مسخن للجسد الحمص الاسود والاحمر اقوى حراره
من الابيض العدس بارد في الدرجه الاولى يابس في الدرجه
الثانيه مظلم للبصر الجاوشير والدخن باردان

17A

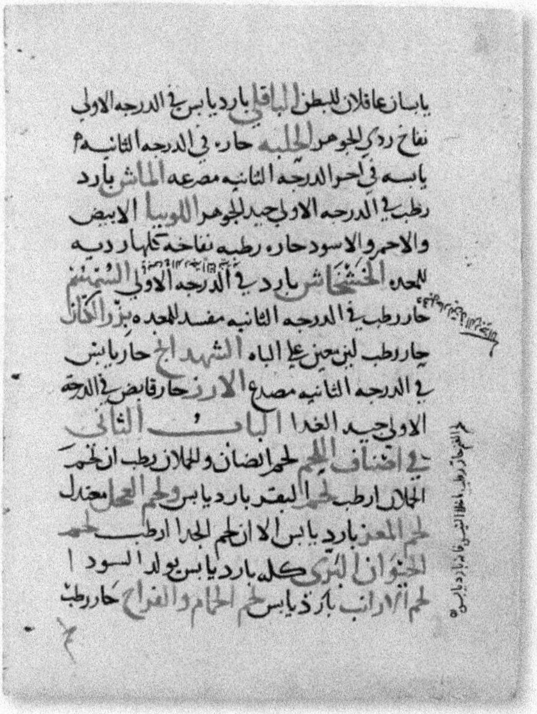
يابسان عاقلان للبطن الباقلي بارد يابس في الدرجه الاولى
نفاخ رديء الجوهر الحلبه حار في الدرجه الثانيه
يابسه في اخر الدرجه الثانيه مصدعه الماش بارد
رطب في الدرجه الاولى جيد الجوهر اللوبيا الابيض
والاحمر والاسود حاره رطبه نفاخه كلها رديه
للمعده الخشخاش بارد في الدرجه الاولى السمسم
حار رطب في الدرجه الثانيه مفسد للمعده بزر الكتان
حار رطب لين معين على الباه الشهدانج حار يابس
في الدرجه الثانيه مصدع الارز حار قابض في الدرجه
الاولى جيد الغدا الباب الثاني
في اصناف اللحم لحم الضان والحملان رطب ان لحم
الحملان ارطب لحم البقر بارد يابس ولحم العجل معتدل
لحم المعز بارد يابس الا ان لحم الجداء ارطب لحم
الحيوان البري كله بارد يابس يولد السودا
لحم الارانب بارد يابس لحم الحمام والفراخ حار رطب

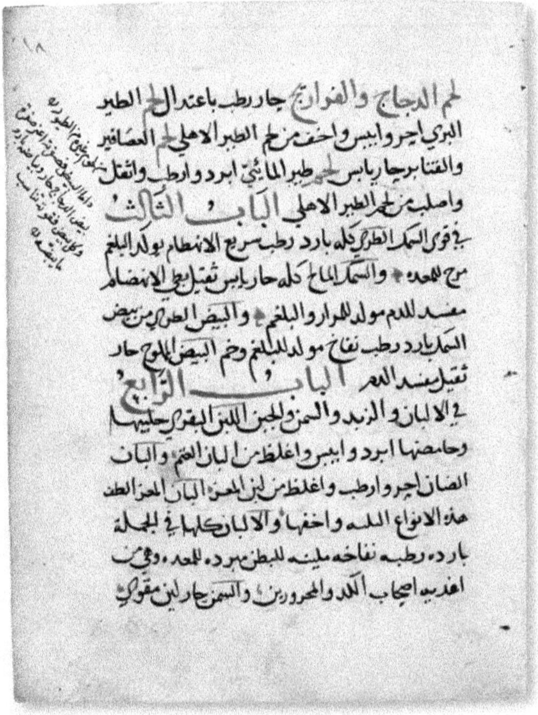

١٨

لحم الدجاج والفراريج حار رطب باعتدال لحم الطير
البري احر وايبس واخف من لحم الطير الاهلي لحم العصافير
والقنابر حار يابس لحم طير المائي ابرد وارطب واثقل
واصلب من لحم الطير الاهلي

الباب الثالث

في قوى السمك الطري كله بارد رطب سريع الانهضام يولد البلغم
مرخ للمعده ٭ والسمك المالح كله حار يابس ثقيل بطي الانهضام
مفسد للدم مولد للمرار والبلغم ٭ والبيض الطري من بيض
السمك بارد رطب نفاخ مولد للبلغم وخم البيض المملوح حار
ثقيل مفسد للدم

الباب الرابع

في الالبان والزبد والسمن والجبن اللبن البقري حليبها
وحامضها ابرد وايبس واغلظ من البان الغنم والبان
الضان احر وارطب واغلظ من لبن المعز والبان المعز الطف
هذه الانواع الثلاثه واخفها والالبان كلها في الجملة
بارده رطبه نفاخه مليينه للبطن مبرده للمعده وهي من
اغذية اصحاب الكد والمحرورين والسمن حار لين مقوي

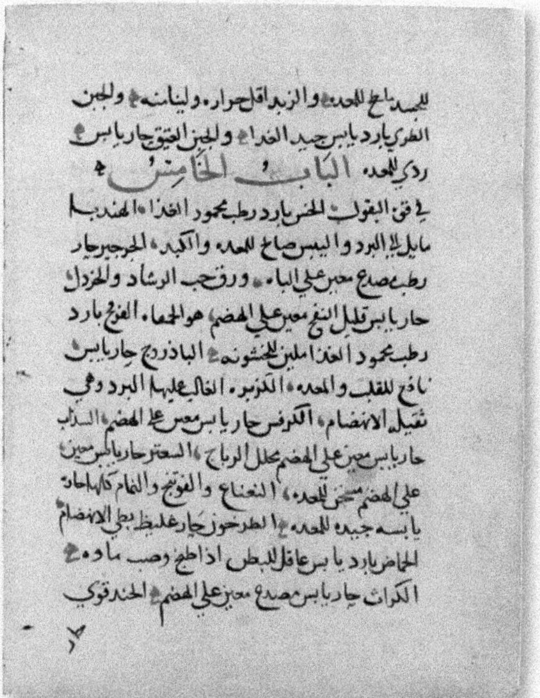
للجسد صالح للمعده والزبد اقل حرارة وليانه والجبن
الطري بارد يابس جيد الغذا والجبن العتيق حار يابس
ردي للمعده الباب الخامس
في قوى البقول الخس بارد رطب محمود الغذا الهندبا
مايل الى البرد واليبس صالح للمعده والكبد الجرجير حار
رطب مصدع معين على الباه وورق حب الرشاد والخردل
حار يابس قليل النفع معين على الهضم هو الحما الفرفخ بارد
رطب محمود الغذا ملين للخشونه الباذروج حار يابس
نافع للقلب والمعده الكزبره الغالب عليها البرد وهي
ثقيله الانهضام الكرفس حار يابس معين على الهضم السذاب
حار يابس معين على الهضم محلل الرياح السعتر حار يابس معين
على الهضم مسخن للمعده النعناع والفوتنج والنمام كلها حاره
يابسه جيده للمعده الطرخون حار غليظ بطي الانهضام
الحماض بارد يابس عاقل للبطن اذا طبخ وصب ماوه
الكراث حار يابس مصدع معين على الهضم الخندقوقي

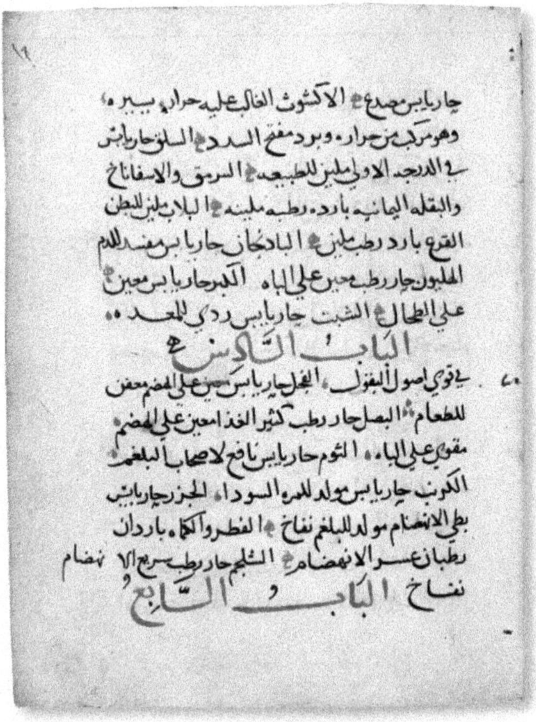

١٩

جار يابس مصدع ه الاكشوث الغالب عليه حرارة ببرده
وهو مركب من حرارة وبرد مفتح السدد ه السلق حار يابس
في الدرجة الاولى ملين للطبيعة ه السرمق والاسفاناخ
والبقلة اليمانية باردة رطبة ملينة ه اللبلاب ملين للبطن
القرع بارد رطب ملين ه الباذنجان حار يابس مفسد للدم
الهليون حار رطب معين على الباه ه الكبر حار يابس معين
على الطحال ه الشبت حار يابس ردي للمعدة ه

الباب السادس

في قوي اصول البقول ه الفجل حار يابس معين على الهضم معفن ٢٠
للطعام ه البصل حار رطب كثير الغذا معين على الهضم
مقوي على الباه ه الثوم حار يابس نافع لاصحاب البلغم
الكرنب حار يابس مولد للمرة السوداء ه الجزر حار يابس
بطي الانهضام مولد للبلغم نفاخ ه الفطر والكماه باردان
رطبان عسر الانهضام ه الشلجم حار رطب سريع الانهضام
نفاخ

الباب السابع

في قوى الفاكهة الرطبة الرمان الحامض بارد يابس عاقل للطبيعة
الرمان الحلو معتدل وخاصة الاملبيسي فانه لطيف مطفي
التفاح الحلو معتدل الحرارة و الحامض بارد وكلاهما
عاقل للطبيعة مقوى للمعدة الخوخ بارد رطب غليظ مولد
للبلغم المشمش بارد رطب مولد للرطوبات التوت الابيض
معتدل البرد والاسود معتدل الحرارة والاحمر منه بارد
وكلاهما عاقل للطبيعة الا ان احلاه اقل بردا وعقلا
للطبيعة العنب الاسود الحلو حار رطب بطي الانهضام
نفاخ مطلق للطبيعة والابيض اقل حرارة وجميع اصناف
التمر والرطب حارة رطبة مصدعة مرخية للمعدة
مولدة للدم الغزير وجميع اصناف البسر حارة
يابسة عاقل للبطن بطي الانهضام التين الرطب حار
رطب على قدر حلاوته ملين الطبيعة الاجاص الحلو
بارد رطب مطلق للبطن والحامض منه ابرد واقل اطلاقا
الموز معتدل في قوته على قدر صنعه وهو حار رطب

قصب السكر حار رطب لطيف باعتدال نافع للصدر
الزعرور بارد يابس عاقل للبطن البنو مثله البطيخ
الحلو سريع الانهضام والاستحاله الي المرار وغير الحلو
بارد سريع الاستحاله الي البلغم القثا والخيار باردان
رطبان مولدان للبلغم والرياح وبزرهما مدر البول

الباب الثامن

في قوي الفاكهه اليابسه العناب معتدل الحراره ملطف
للدم السبستان بارد رطب ملين الصدر اللوز حار
لين باعتدال اللوز الرطب بارد رطب غليظ نفاخ
الفستق حار يابس البندق معتدل في الحر واليبس
عاقل للبطن الجوز اليابس حار يابس والرطب اقل
حراره وبساوفيه نفخ وثقل الغبيرا بارده يابسه
عاقله للبطن الخوخ المقدد معتدل في الحر والبرد
مولد للبلغم المشمش المقدد قوته علي قدر حلاوته
وحموضته والحلو منه مايل الي الحراره والحامض منه

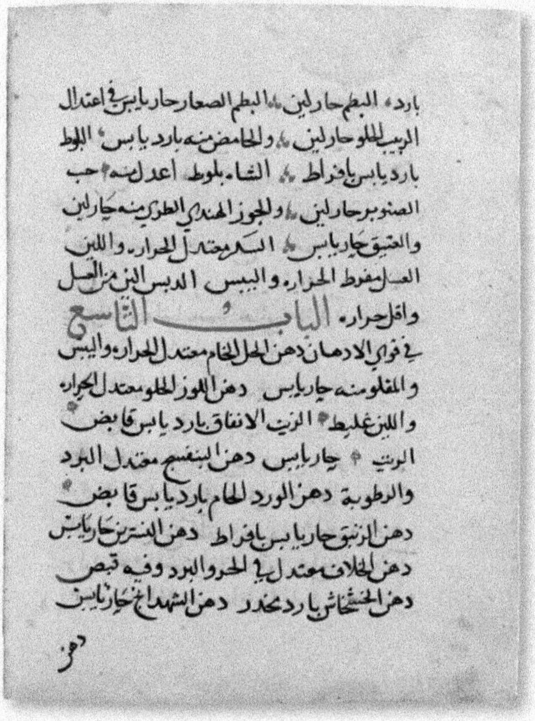

بارد ٭ البطم حار لين ٭ البطم الصغار حار يابس في اعتدال
الزبيب الحلو حار لين ٭ والحامض منه بارد يابس ٭ البلوط
بارد يابس بافراط ٭ الشاه بلوط اعدل منه ٭ حب
الصنوبر حار لين ٭ والجوز الهندي الطري منه حار لين
والعتيق حار يابس ٭ السكر معتدل الحرارة واللين
العسل مفرط الحرارة واليبس الدبس الين من العسل
واقل حرارة

الباب التاسع

في قوى الادهان دهن الحل الخام معتدل الحرارة واليبس
والمقلو منه حار يابس دهن اللوز الحلو معتدل الحرارة
واللين غليظ ٭ الزيت الانفاق بارد يابس قابض
الزيت ٭ حار يابس دهن البنفسج معتدل البرد
والرطوبة دهن الورد الخام بارد يابس قابض
دهن الزنبق حار يابس بافراط دهن النسرين حار يابس
دهن الخلاف معتدل في الحر والبرد وفيه قبض
دهن الخشخاش بارد مخدر دهن الشهدانج حار يابس

دهن

21

دهن النيلوفر بارد لين دهن جار يابس دهن البان
حار يابس دهن الخردل حار يابس دهن الفستق
حار لين للخيري معتدل في الحر والبرد دهن تفاح
الحيار بارد قابض دهن البابونج حار لين دهن
المرزجوش حار يابس الباب العاشر
في فعل الرياحين الورد مركب القوة قابض السوسن
الازاد حار يابس النرجس حار لين البنفسج حار لين
النيلوفر بارد يابس النمام حار يابس النسرين
معتدل الحرارة الشاهسفرم في اول الحرارة معتدل
الحرارة واذا ابرز كان حار ايابسا الحماحم حار يابس
الفلنجمشك حار يابس في اعتدال الحرارة المرماحوز
حار يابس والشيح والقيصوم حاران يابسان اللفاح
مركب القوة مخدر تفاح الخلاف معتدل في الحرارة
والبرد الياسمين الاخضر حار يابس والابيض
معتدل والاصفر ضعيف القوة والاس مركب القوة

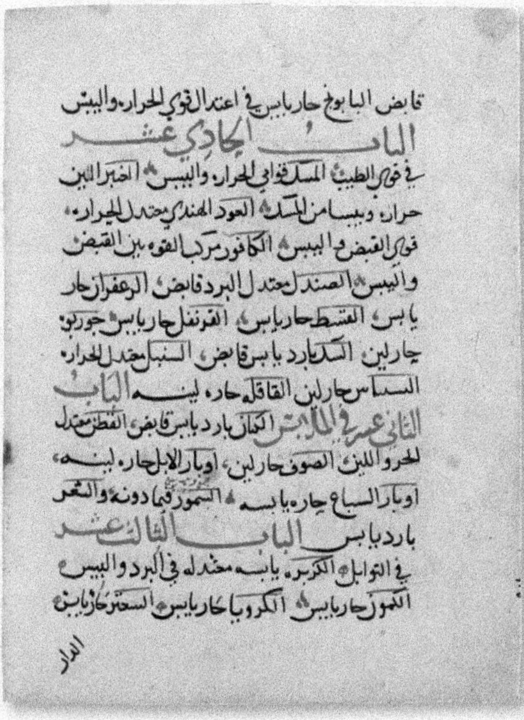

قابض البابونج حار يابس في اعتدال قوي الحرارة واليبس
الباب الحادي عشر
في قوى الطيب المسك قوي الحرارة واليبس العنبر لين
حار ويبسا من المسك العود الهندي معتدل الحرارة
قوي القبض واليبس الكافور مركب القوة بين القبض
واليبس الصندل معتدل البرد قابض الزعفران حار
يابس القسط حار يابس القرنفل حار يابس جوزبوا
حار لين السك بارد يابس قابض السنبل معتدل الحرارة
السناس حار لين القاقلة حارة لينة الباب
الثاني عشر في الملابس الكتان بارد يابس قابض القطن معتدل
الحر واللين الصوف حار لين اوبار الابل حارة لينة
اوبار السباع حارة يابسة السمور فيما دونه والشعر
بارد يابس الباب الثالث عشر
في التوابل الكزبرة يابسة معتدلة في البرد واليبس
الكمون حار يابس الكرويا حار يابس السعتر حار يابس
الدار

الدارصيني يابس جدا معتدل الحراره • الزنجبيل والخولنجان
حاران يابسان • النانخوه قويه الحراره واليبس •
الشونيز قوي الحراره واليبس • الخردل قوي الحراره واليبس
الانجدان والحلتيت المحروق حاران يابسان • الكاشم
معتدل الحراره واليبس • السماق بارد يابس • الابرنا يس
مركب القوه معتدل لطيف • الابهل حار يابس • الملح حار يابس

الباب الرابع عشر •

في الخل والمري والزيتون والكوامخ والرواصير • الخل
بارد لطيف • المري حار يابس • الكوامخ قوتها على قدر ما
يتخذ منه وهي كلها رديه للمعده معطشه مفسده
للدم • قضبان الكبر المربا بالخل ملطفه جيده للطحال
الثوم المربا بالخل معين على الهضم ناقص الحراره لاسيما
العتيق منه • المتخذ بالقبول الحاره • المرسين ناقص
البرد والنفخ • والماسسع بارد رطب • المصل بارد
يابس • الكرفس الجبلي المربا بالخل حار لطيف معين على الهضم والمنو

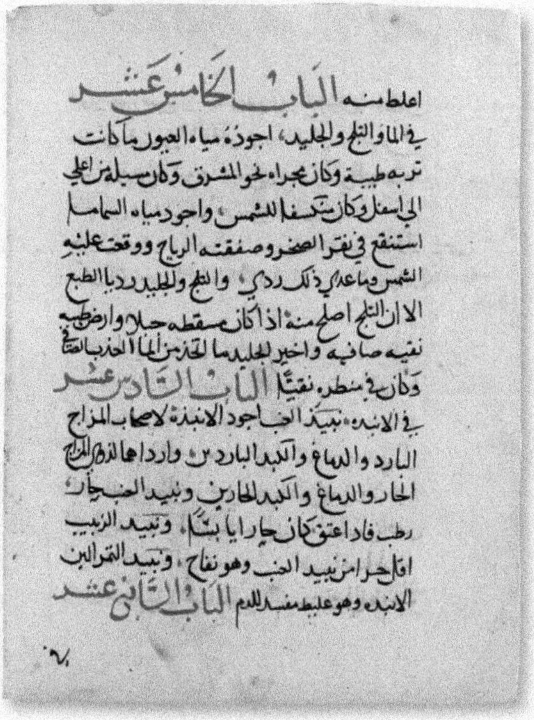

اعلط منه الباب الخامس عشر
في الما والثلج والجليد، اجوده مياه العيون ما كانت
تربه طيبة وكان مجراه نحو المشرق وكان سيله من اعلى
الى اسفل وكان متكشفا للشمس، واجود مياه السما ما
استنقع في نقر الصخر وصفقته الرياح ووقعت عليه
الشمس وما عدا ذلك ردي، والثلج والجليد رديا الطبع
الا ان الثلج اصلح منه اذا كان مسقطه جبلا وارضا طيبه
نقيه صافيه واخير الجليد ما اتخذ من الما العذب الصافي
وكان في سطح نقيا الباب السادس عشر
في الانبذه، نبيذ العنب اجود الانبذه لاصحاب المزاج
البارد والدماغ والكبد البارد من واردا ها للذي المزاج
الحار والدماغ والكبد الحارين ونبيذ العنب حار
رطب فاذا عتق كان حارا يابسا، ونبيذ الزبيب
اقل حرا من نبيذ العنب وهو نفاخ، ونبيذ التمر الين
الانبذه وهو غليظ مفسد للدم الباب السابع عشر

٩٧

في الاشربه والربوب السكنجبين الساذج بارد لطيف
والمتخذ منه بالاصول والبزور حار وهو انفع للمعده والكبد
الحارين من الساذج والاسكنجبين يضعف المعده والصعب
كله لحموضته والجلاب معتدل الحراره نافع للمعده اذا شرب
من مزاج قليل شراب البنفسج معتدل في الحر والبرد
ملين للبطن مرخ للمعده المتيبة المركبة بالافا وبه صلاحة
للمعده حابس للبطن والساذج اصلح للمحرورين رب
السفرجل ورب التفاح بارد ان عاقلان للبطن رب
الحصرم ابرد من ذلك وهو حابس للبطن مسكن للعطش
رب الرمان جيد للمعده مسكن للغثيان رب التوث
بارد مطلق للطبيعه صالح لبثور الفم ووجع الحلق

الباب الثامن عشر

في الانبجات الجلنجبين السكري مقوي للمعده مسخن لها
والعسلي اقوى حراره من السكري البنفسج المربا معتدل
في الحراره والبرد ملين للصدر والبطن الزنجبيل

23A

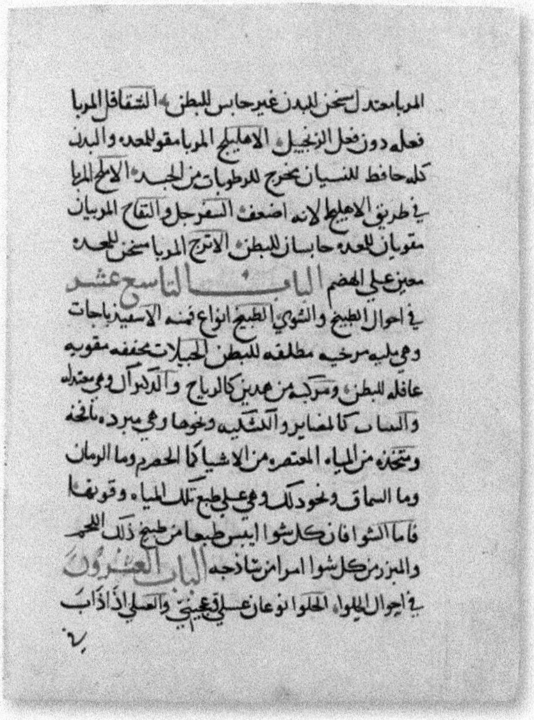

المربا معتدل يسخن للبدن غير حابس للبطن ۞ التشاقل المربا
فعله دون فعل الزنجبيل ۞ الاهليلج المربا مقو للمعده والبدن
كله حافظ للنسيان يخرج للرطوبات من الجسد ۞ الاملج المربا
في طريق الاهليلج لانه اضعف ۞ السفرجل والتفاح المربيان
مقويان للمعده حابسان للبطن ۞ الاترج المربا يسخن للمعده
معين على الهضم الباب التاسع عشر
في احوال الطبيخ والشوي الطبيخ انواع فمنه الاسفيذباجات
وهي مليه مرخيه مطلقه للبطن الجبلات محففه مقويه
عاقله للبطن ۞ ومركبه من هذين كالرباج والدكبراك وهي معتدله
والنماب كالمضاير والكشكيه ونحوها وهي مبرده نافخه
ومتخذه من المياه المعتصره من الاشيا كالحصرم وما الرمان
وما السماق ونحو ذلك وهي على طبع تلك المياه وقوتها
فاما الشوا فان كل شوا ايبس طبعا من طبيخ ذلك اللحم
والمبزر من كل شوا امرا من ناذجه الباب العشرون
في احوال الحلوا الحلوا نوعان عسلي وعجيني والعسلي اذا ذاب
٤٧

في الفم وصار الى المعده اعان على الهضم ولين الطبيعه فان
كان مربب باللوزدان وخما ثقيلا متخما واما العجيني
فغليظ بطي الانهضام مولد للسدد في العروق والمفاصل
والحلوا كله كثير الغذا مكثر للدم ويعين على الباه تمت المقاله
الثانيه

المقاله الثالثه

في حفظ الصحه وتربيه الطفل وتدبير الحبلي وهي عشره ابواب

الباب الاول منها

في الحركات الرياضيه القويه الكامله للجسد هي المصارعه
ودونها العدو ودونها الركض ودونها المشي فاما الخاصيه
فان القراه بصوت عال تحرك الراس وما فيه من الاعضا
فتسخنه وتنقيه وتسده القوه وتعده لقبول الغذا
ورفع الحجر والنزع في القسي الصلبه والضرب واللعب بالصو
لجان والكره وخاصه الكبيره تحرك البدن والعنق والصدر
والكتف والظهر فتسخنها وتقويها وتنقيها والمشي السريع
تحرك الاليتين والفخذين والساقين والقدمين فتسخنها

وتقويها واعدل الحركات الرياضيه المشي الرفيق والحركة
تثير الحراره الغريزيه وتنبهها والسكون يخمد الحراره
الغريزيه ويطفيها الباب الثاني
في الحمام ينبغي ان يكون فسيح الهوا عذب الما وان يسخن
بالحطب ولا يسخن بالسرجين فان هوا الحمام انما هو من
بخار ما يوقد به الاتون فان كان الوقود جيدا كان بخاره
جيدا وان كان رديا كان بخاره رديا فينبغي ان
يكون هوا الحمام غير مفرط الحراره ولا لين الحراره جدا
فان الاول يلجي العرق على الخروج ويحمي القلب ويصدع
والثاني لا يحدث العرق ولا البخار ويستعمل في كل بيت
من البيوت الحمام ما يشاكله من الما وان لا يستعمل في البيت
الحار الما البارد ولا في البيت البارد الما الشديد الحراره
فان ذلك يحدث الاقشعرار ويسد خروق الجسد ومسامه
وينبغي ان يكون دخول الابزن بعد لبث في هوا
الحمام وتعديله الجسد بالما وان لا يطيل الانسان الجلوس

من الابزن

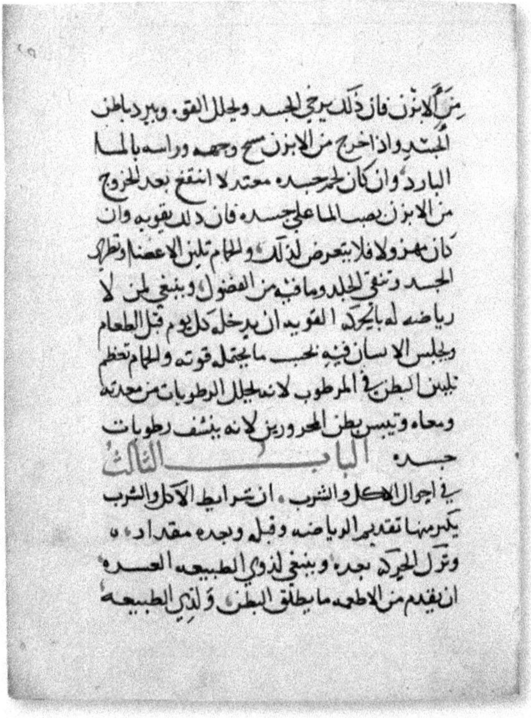

٢٩

من الابزن فان ذلك يرخي الجسد ويحلل القوى ويبرد باطن
الجسد واذا اخرج من الابزن مسح وجهه وراسه بالما
البارد وان كان لحم جسده معتدلا انتفع بعد الخروج
من الابزن بصب الما على جسده فان ذلك يقويه وان
كان مهزولا فلا يتعرض لذلك وللحمام تلين الاعضا وتطرى
الجسد وتنقي الجلد وما فيه من الفضول وينبغي لمن لا
رياضة له بالحركة القوية ان يدخله كل يوم قبل الطعام
ويجلس الانسان فيه بحسب ما يحتمله قوته وللحمام تعظم
تليين البطن في المرطوب لانه يحلل الرطوبات من معدته
ومعاه وتيبس بطن المحرورين لانه ينشف رطوبات
جسده

الباب الثالث

في احوال الاكل والشرب ان شرايط الاكل والشرب
يكثر منها تقديم الرياضة وقبله وبعده مقدار
وترك الحركة بعده وينبغي لذوي الطبيعة العسرة
ان يقدم من الاطعمة ما يطلق البطن ولذي الطبيعة

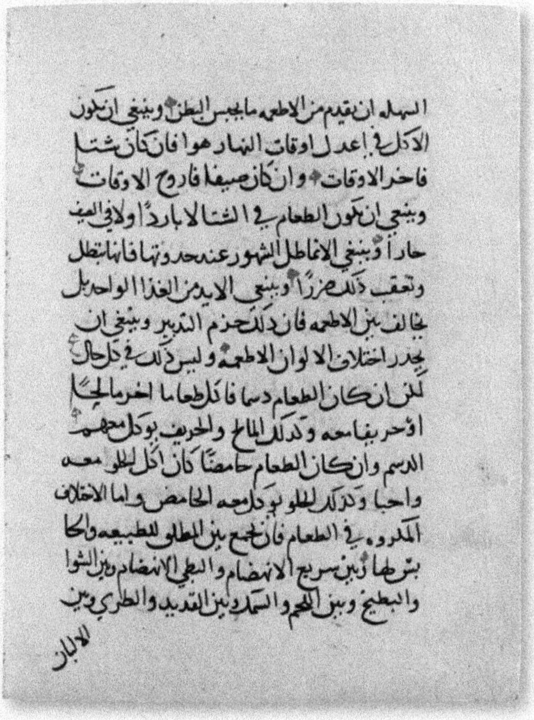

السهله ان يقدم من الاطعمه ما يحبس البطن وينبغي ان يكون
الاكل في اعدل اوقات النهار هوا فان كان شتا
فاخر الاوقات وان كان صيفا فاروح الاوقات
وينبغي ان يكون الطعام في الشتا لا باردا ولا في الصيف
حارا وينبغي الا ماطل الشهوه عند حدوثها فانها تبطل
وتعقب ذلك ضررا وينبغي الا يدمن الغذا الواحد بل
يخالف بين الاطعمه فان ذلك حزم التدبير وينبغي ان
يحذر اختلاف الالوان الاطعمه وليس ذلك في كل حال
لكن ان كان الطعام دسما فاكل طعاما اخر ما لحا
او حريفا معه وكذلك المالح والحريف يوكل معهم
الدسم وان كان الطعام حامضا كان اكل الحلو معه
واجبا وكذلك الحلو يوكل معه الحامض واما الاختلاف
المكروه في الطعام فان يجمع بين المطلق للطبيعه والحا
بس لها وبين سريع الانهضام والبطي الانهضام وبين الشوا
والطبيخ وبين اللحم والسمك وبين القديد والطري وبين
الالبان

الالبان واللحوم وبين البيض واللحم وبين البقل والسمك
واما السرات فوجه تسكين العطش على الطعام وبعده
وحده الا يغلب على الطعام حتى يجعله طافيا ويحول بينه وبين
جرم المعده ان تحتوي عليه ويجوز مقدار برده الا يبين على
الاسنان ولا على الاحشا برده حاما الما الفاتر فلا خير
فيه

الباب الرابع

في النوم واليقظه . النوم يريح الاعضا ويهضم الطعام
ويجم النفس ويجلب افعال الطبيعه في البدن والافرا ط
منه يبرد الجسد ويبلد النفس ويهيج الوجه واما السهر
فيبس الجسد وينقي رطوباته ويحلل القوى ويمنع من الاستمرا
ويفسد المزاج والافراط فيه يورث الجنون

الباب الخامس في احوال الباه

دليل الحاجه الى الباه هو الشهوه اليه على بعد العهد به
فاما على قرب العهد فلا وتركها في تلك الحال يضجر
النفس ويبطل شهوه الطعام ويحول بين الجسد وبين استبقا

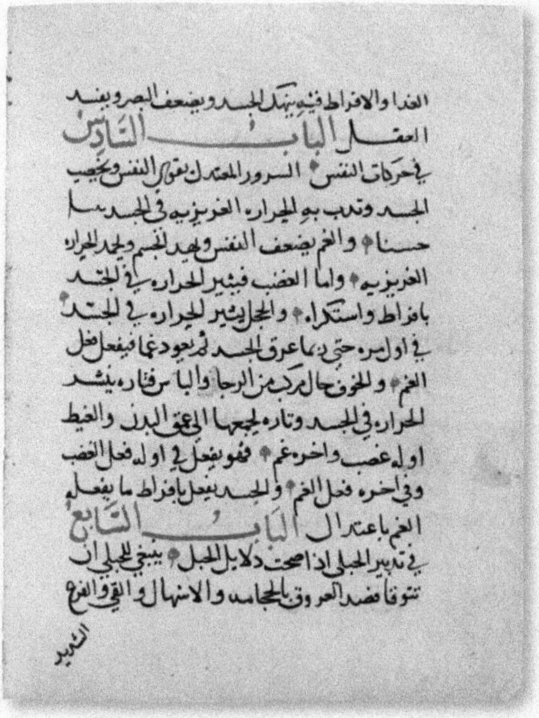

الغذا والافراط فيه ينهك الجسد ويضعف البصر ويفسد
العقل الباب السادس
في حركات النفس ◆ السرور المعتدل يقوي النفس ويخصب
الجسد وتدب به الحراره الغريزيه في الجسد بسلا
حسنا ◆ والغم يضعف النفس ويهد الجسم ويخمد الحراره
الغريزيه ◆ واما الغضب فيثير الحراره في الجسد
بافراط واستكرا ◆ والخجل يثير الحراره في الجسد
في اول امره حتى يدما عرق الجسد ثم يعود غما فيفعل فعل
الغم ◆ وللخوف حال مركب من الرجا والياس فتاره ينشر
الحراره في الجسد وتاره يجمعها الى عمق البدن والغيظ
اوله غضب واخره غم ◆ فهو يفعل في اوله فعل الغضب
وفي اخره فعل الغم ◆ والحسد يفعل بافراط ما يفعله
الغم باعتدال الباب السابع
في تدبير الحبلى اذا صحت دلايل الحبل ◆ ينبغي للحبلى ان
تتوقا فصد العروق والحجامه والاسهال والقي والفزع
التدبير

٢٧

الشديد والاصوات الهايله وشم الروايح القويه من روايح
الاطعمه الى ان ياتي عليها اربعه اشهر فان الح بها الامر
بعد ذلك الى فصد او حجامة او اسهال فليستعمل ذلك
ان كانت قويه الجسد غير خفيفه الى ان تجاوز الشهر
السابع ثم تمسك ايضا عن ذلك وتحذره • وينبغي للحبلى ان
تكثر العنايه بفم المعده حتى لا تشتهي التطين والاشيا
الرديه تتعاهد بالحلنجبين والاسكنجبين الممزوج الجيد

الباب الثامن

في تدبير المرضعه • ليس يجوز للمرضعه ان ترضع الطفل
وزوجها ينتاب فراشها فان ذلك يفسد لبنها ويمرض
الطفل وهو الغيل الذي كرهته العرب • وينبغي ان تاكل
غذا من اجود الاغذيه وابعدها من الفساد • وان
تتحرك فضل حركه وتروض جسدها ولا تلزم الدعة
والسكون فان ذلك يفسد لبنها

الباب التاسع

في تدبير الطفل الى بلوغه • تدبير الطفل ما دام رضيعا

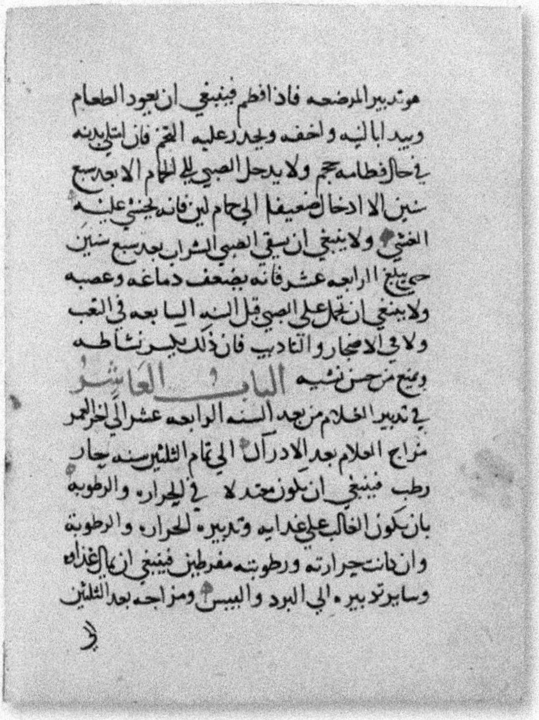

هو تدبير المرضعه فاذا افطم فينبغي ان يعود الطعام
ويبدا بالنيه واخفه ويحذر عليه التخم فان اشتكي بدنه
في حال فطامه حجم ولا يدخل الصبي الي الحمام الا بعد سبع
سنين الا ادخالا ضعيفا الي حمام لين فانه يخشي عليه
الغشي ولا ينبغي ان يسقي الصبي الشراب بعد سبع سنين
حتي يبلغ الرابعه عشر فانه يضعف دماغه وعصبه
ولا ينبغي ان يحمل علي الصبي قبل السنه السابعه في التعب
ولا في الاضجار والتاديب فان ذلك يكسر نشاطه
ويمنع من حسن نشئه الباب العاشر
في تدبير الغلام من بعد السنه الرابعه عشر الي اخر العمر
مزاج الغلام بعد الادراك الي تمام الثلثين سنه حار
رطب فينبغي ان يكون معتدلا في الحراره والرطوبه
بان يكون الغالب علي غذايه وتدبيره الحراره والرطوبه
وان كانت حرارته ورطوبته مفرطين فينبغي ان يميل غذاه
وساير تدبيره الي البرد واليبس ومزاجه بعد الثلثين
الي

27B

٢٠٦

الي مجاوره بعد الثلثين الي مجاوزه الاربعين حار يابس
فان حرارته ويبسه معتدلين فينبغي ان تكون الغالب
علي غذايه وتدبيره الحر واليبس المعتدلين وان
كانا مفرطين فينبغي ان يمال غذاوه وتدبيره الي البرد
والرطوبه ومزاجه بعد الاربعين الي الستين بارد
يابس فان كان في ذلك معتدلا ان يكون غذاو
وتدبيره معتدلا في الحر واليبس وان كان يجاوز
الاعتدال فينبغي ان يمال الغذا والتدبير الي
الحراره والرطوبه ومزاجه بعد الستين الي اخر
العمر يكون مختلفا لان اعضاه بارده يابسه والرطوبه
البلغميه في تجاويف اعضايه كثيره فينبغي ان
يدبر بحسب الاغلب مما ذكرنا. تمت المقاله الثالثه
بعون الله وحسن توفيقه

المقاله الرابعه

في امراض الراس وهي ثمنيه عشر بابا

الباب الاول في الصداع والشقيقه

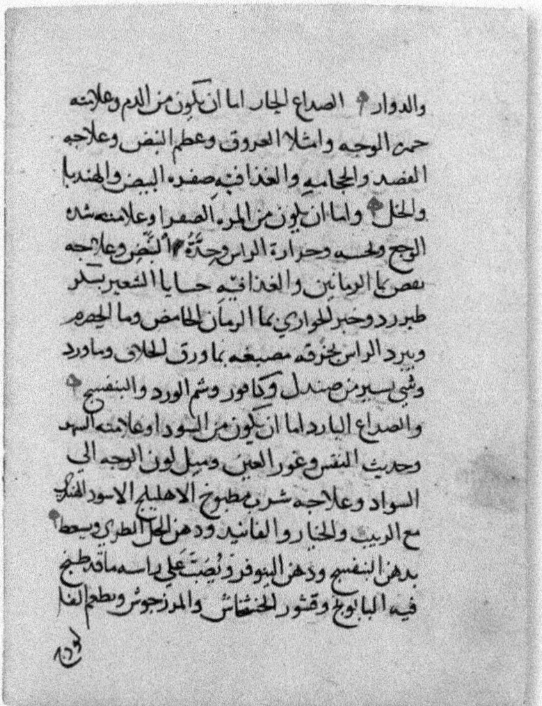
والدوار ❁ الصداع الحار اما ان يكون من الدم وعلامته
حمرة الوجه وامتلا العروق وعظم النبض وعلاجه
الفصد والحجامة والغذا فيه صفرة البيض والهندبا
والخل ❁ واما ان يكون من المرة الصفرا وعلامته شدة
الوجع والحسه وحرارة الراس وحدة النبض وعلاجه
نقص بما الرمانين والغذا فيه حسايا الشعير بسكر
طبرزد وخبز الحواري بما الرمان الحامض وما الحصرم
ويبرد الراس بخرقه مصبغه بما ورق الخلاف وماورد
وشي يسير من صندل وكافور وشم الورد والبنفسج ❁
والصداع البارد اما ان يكون من السودا وعلامته السهر
وحديث النفس وغور العين وميل لون الوجه الي
السواد وعلاجه شرب مطبوخ الاهليلج الاسود المنكى(?)
مع الزبيب والخيار والفانيد ودهن الخل الطري ويسعط ❁
بدهن البنفسج ودهن النيلوفر ويصب علي راسه ماقد طبخ
فيه البابونج وقشور الخشخاش والمرزجوش ويطعم الغذا
لحوم(?)

٢٩

لوج ويتغذا ايام بالفراريج زيرباج • واما ان يكون
الصداع من البلغم العفن وعلامته ثقل الراس وتهيج
الوجه وعلاجه سقي حب الايارج وحب الشبيار د
ويسعط بدهن الخيري • ودهن البابونج ويستعمل شم
المرزنجوش والنرجس ويطعم العصافير والقنابر
وهكذا علاج الشقيقة تخص الجانب العليل بالسعوط
وهكذا علاج الدوار الا انه يستعمل في الدوار •
والشقيقة والقي بعد الاكلات

الباب الثاني

في السرسام الحار • السرسام الحار اما ان يكون من
الدم واما ان يكون من الصفرا فما كان من الدم فعلامته
حمرة الوجه وعظم النبض وحمرة البول وخفة اختلاط
العقل وملازمة الحمى • وعلاجه سقي ما الشعير مع شراب
العناب • فاذا افاق العليل غذي بالخبز الحواري المثرو ل
بالشيرين السكر الطبرزد وبعد ذلك مزوره العدس
المقشر ودهن اللوز والخل اياما • وان كان من المرة

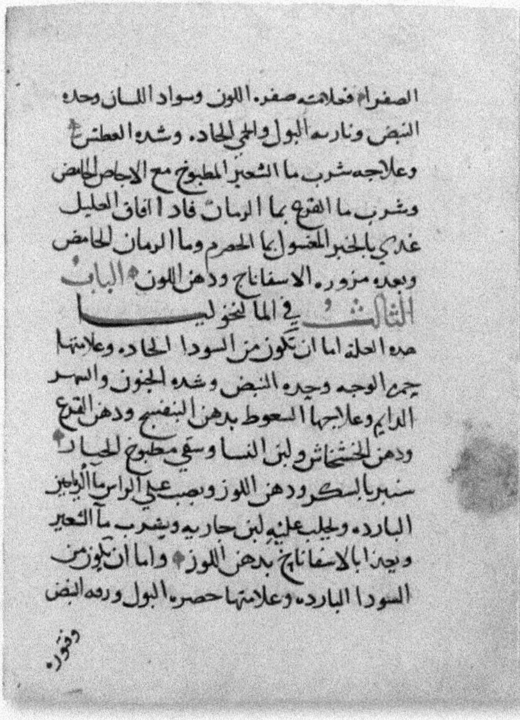
الصفرا فعلامته صفره اللون وسواد اللسان وحده
النبض ونارسه البول والحمى الحاد. وشده العطش
وعلاجه شرب ما الشعير المطبوخ مع الاجاص الحامض
وشرب ما القرع بما الرمان فاد ا افاق العليل
غذي بالخبز المغسول بما الحصرم وما الرمان الحامض
وبعده مزوره الاسفاناج ودهن اللوز. الباب
الثالث في الماليخوليا
هذه العلة اما ان تكون من السودا الحاده وعلامتها
حمرة الوجه وحده النبض وشده الجنون والسهر
الدايم وعلاجها السعوط بدهن البنفسج ودهن القرع
ودهن الخشخاش ولبن النسا وسقي مطبوخ الحياد
شنبر بالسكر ودهن اللوز ويصب علي الراس ما الرياحين
البارده ويحلب عليه لبن جاريه ويشرب ما الشعير
ويغذا بالاسفاناخ بدهن اللوز. واما ان تكون من
السودا البارده وعلامتها حصره البول ورقه النبض
وفتوره

وفتوره وهدوا العليل وعلاجها صب ما الرياحين الحاره
على الراس والسعوط بدهن الحل او دهن الاكارع ويحلب
على الراس من لبن النسا وسقي العليل مطبوخ الافتيمون
ويطعم الفراريج بالما لوذج الرقيق ويدخل الحمام وان
كان عريا ووح

الباب الرابع في الصرع

ان كان من البلغم فعلامته بياض اللون
وخصب البدن ويقدم اكل الاغذيه البلغميه
عولج بحب الارياج وحب القوقايا واطعم الطير
البري شوا ومطبوخا مطجنا ومزج ماء بالسكنجبين
العسلي وان كان معه علامه السودا وهي الهزال
وسواد اللون وقذف المره السودا الحامضه في
وقت الصرع عولج بمطبوخ الافتيمون والاغاريقون
وبايارج دوفر ولطف غذاء وسقي الشراب

الباب الخامس في العشق

اذا احدث من العشق الجهد والسهر والهزال الخشي على صاحبه

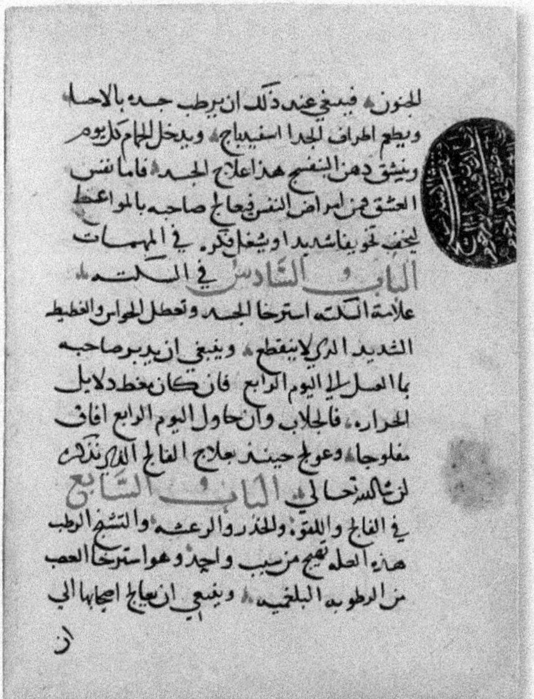

للجنون فينبغي عند ذلك ان يرطب جسده بالاحسا
ويطعم اطراف الجدا اسفيدباج ويدخل الحمام كل يوم
ويستنشق دهن البنفسج هذا علاج الجسد فاما نفس
العشق من امراض النفس فيعالج صاحبه بالمواعظ
ليخيف تخويفا شديدا او يشغل فكره في المهمات

الباب السادس في السكته

علامة السكته استرخا الجسد وتعطل الحواس والغطيط
الشديد الذي لا ينقطع وينبغي ان يدبر صاحبه
بالعسل الى اليوم الرابع فان كان فقط دلايل
الحراره فالجلاب وان جاوز اليوم الرابع افاق
مفلوجا وعولج حينئذ بعلاج الفالج الذي نذكره
ان شا الله تعالى

الباب السابع

في الفالج واللقوه والخدر والرعشه والتشنج الرطب
هذه العله تهيج من سبب واحد وهو استرخا العصب
من الرطوبه البلغميه وينبغي ان يعالج اصحابها الي
ان

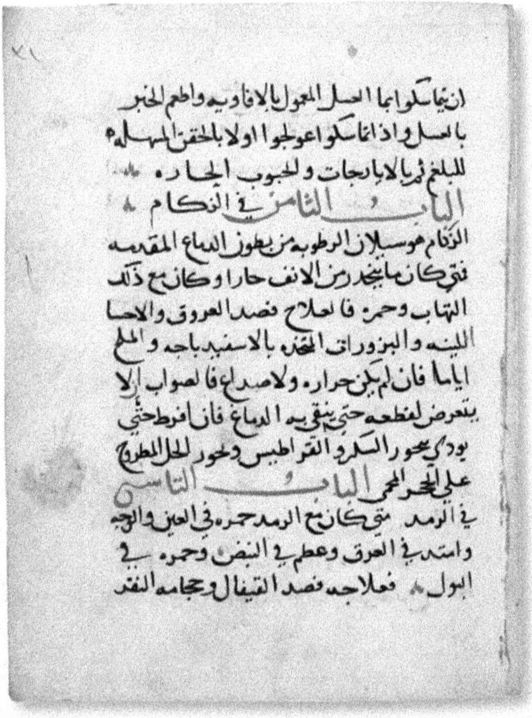

٢١

ان تماسكوا انما العسل المعمول بالافاويه واطعم الخبز
بالعسل واذا تماسكوا عولجوا اولا بالحقن المسهله
للبلغم ثم بالايارجات والحبوب الحاره

الباب الثامن في الزكام

الزكام هو سيلان الرطوبه من بطون الدماغ المقدمه
متى كان ما ينحدر من الانف حارا وكان مع ذلك
التهاب وحمره فالعلاج فصد العروق والاحسا
اللينه والبزورات المحمصه بالاسفيدباجه والملح
اياما فان لم يكن حراره ولا صداع فالصواب ان لا
يتعرض لقطعه حتى ينقى به الدماغ فان افرط حتى
يودي بخور السكر والقراطيس وبخور الخل المطروح
على الحجر المحمى

الباب التاسع

في الرمد متى كان مع الرمد حمره في العين والوجه
وامتلا في العرق وعظم في النبض وحمره في
البول فعلاجه فصد القيفال وحجامه النقره

واسهال الطبيعه بطبيخ الاهليلج الاصفر والخيار شنبر
وبزر القثا ، ويضمد الراس بخرق مصبغه بالماورد
المبرد ، ووضع القدمين في الماء الحار ودلكهما ، والغذا
المزورات المتخذه باللحم والعدس المقشر ودهن اللوز
واكل الخبز بما الحصرم واما الرمان الحامض ومتى كان
مع الرمد ثقله حمره في العين وغلبت دلايل الصفرا
فالعلاج الاسهال بطبيخ الاهليلج والخيار شنبر وتدرك
الفصد ، ويكون الغذا ما قدمنا ذكره ، ومتى لم يكن
في العين حمره وكانت تلتصق في الليل ويكون لها
قذى كثيرا ، فالعلاج لذلك سحق حب الشبيار وفي
كل ليله اولا اياريج فيقرا اسادج ودخول الحمام
في كل يوم وترك العشا وتلطيف الغذا والتغذي
بما الحمص ويدهن الحلق

الباب العاشر

في ضعف البصر وسيلان الدمع ، متى كان ضعف
البصر في حال الكهوله وحال الشيخوخه لم ينفع منه

العلاج

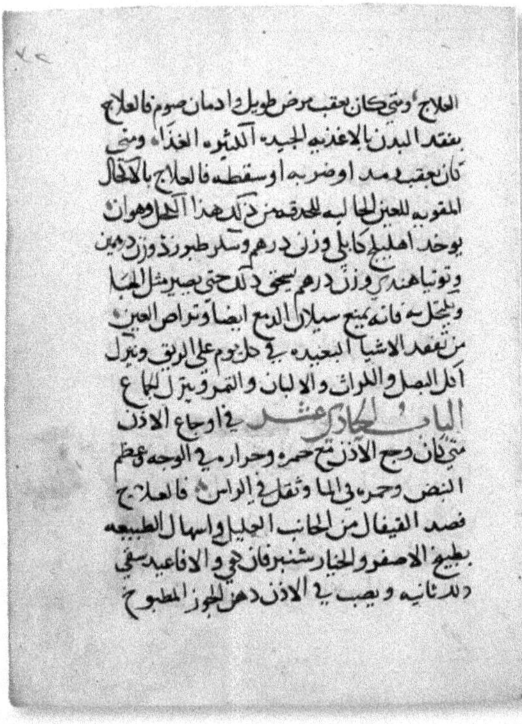

العلاج ومتى كان يعقب مرض طويل وادمان صوم فالعلاج
بتقد البدن بالاغذيه الجيده الكثيره الغذا ومتى
كان يعقب رمد اوضربه او سقطه فالعلاج بالاكحال
المقويه للعين الجاليه للحدقه من ذلك هذا الكحل وهو ان
يوخذ اهليلج كابلي وزن درهم وسكر طبرزذ وزن درهمين
وتوتيا هندي وزن درهم يسحق ذلك حتى يصير مثل الهبا
ويكتحل به فانه يمنع سيلان الدمع ايضا وتراص العين
من تفقد الاشيا البعيده في كل يوم على الريق ويترك
اكل البصل والكراث والالبان والتمر ويترك الجماع
الباب الحادي عشر في اوجاع الاذن
متى كان وجع الاذن مع حمره وحراره في الوجه وعظم
النبض وحمره في الما وثقل في الراس فالعلاج
فصد القيفال من الجانب العليل واسهال الطبيعه
بطبيخ الاصفر والخيار شنبر فان حمي والافاعيد سقي
ذلك ثانيه ويصب في الاذن دهن الجوز المطبوخ

32A

ويكون الغذا المزورات بالعدس والخل والملح ودهن
اللوز، ومتى كان مع وجع الاذن دوي ولس وكان
الوجع يشتد ويهيج ولم يكن في النبض عظم ولا في البول
حمرة. فالعلاج بحب الشيبار وتنقيه المعده
والدماغ والقي والغرغره وبتلطيف الغذا واكل
الزاربا جات بدهن الخل وقطر في الاذن دهن قد
طبخ فيه ورق المرزجوش، ومتى سال من الاذن
مدة بعد الوجع وكان ذلك من انفجار ورم فيها فينبغي
الا تحبس المده حتى يستفرغ عن اخرها فان افرطت
المده فما [illegible] يفرط من تخليط العليل
من ماكول فينبغي ان يحمي العليل وتاخذ فتيلة من خرقة
كتان وتبلها بما الورد وتنثر عليها الكافور وتدسها
في ثقب الاذن

الباب الثاني عشر

في اوجاع الانف، منها نتن المنخرين وينبغي ان تعالج
ذلك بتنقيه المعده بالقي ثم بالاسهال بحب الشيبار

وحر

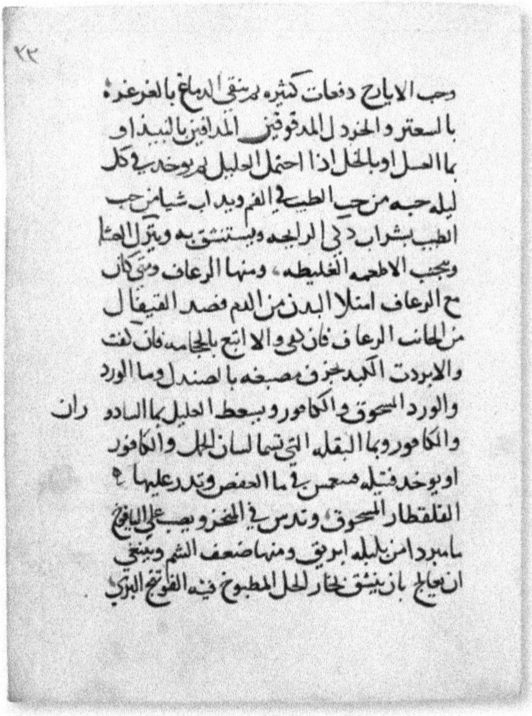

٢٢

وجب الاياج دفعات كثيره ثم ينقى الدماغ بالغرغره
بالسعتر والخردل للمدقوقين المدافين بالنبيذ او
بما العسل او بالخل اذا احتمل العليل ثم يوخذ في كل
ليله حبه من حب الطيب في الفم ويداب شيا من حب
الطيب بشراب ذكي الرايحه ويستنشق به ويترك الامتلا
ويجتنب الاطعمه الغليظه ، ومنها الرعاف ومتى كان
مع الرعاف امتلا البدن من الدم فصد القيفال
من الجانب الرعاف فان دعي والا اتبع بالحجامه فان كنت
والا بردت الكبد بخرق مصبغه بالصندل وما الورد
والورد المسحوق والكافور وبعط العليل بما السادو رات
والكافور وبما البقله التي تسما لسان الحمل والكافور
او يوخذ فتيله مغمس في ما العفص وتذر عليها
القلقطار المسحوق وتدس في المنخر ويصب على اليافوخ
ما مبردا من بلبله ابريق ومنها ضعف الشم وينبغي
ان يعالج بان ينشق بخار الخل المطبوخ فيه القوتنج البري

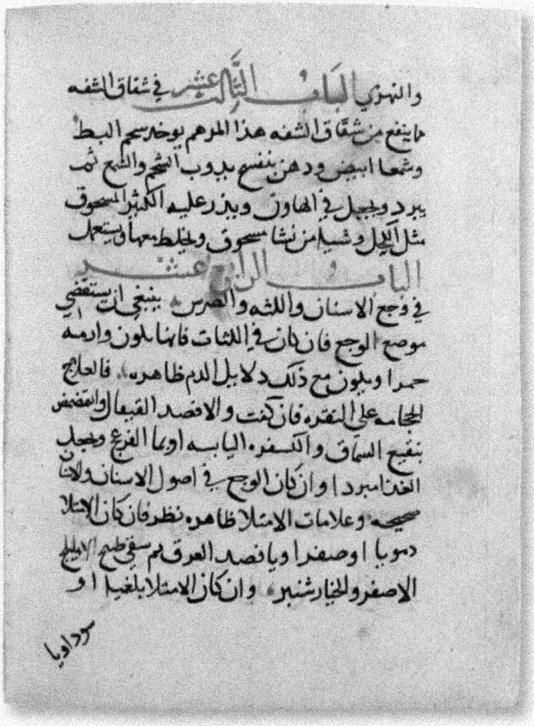

والنهري الباب الثالث عشر في شقاق الشفه
ما ينفع من شقاق الشفه هذا المرهم يوخذ شحم البط
وشمعا ابيض ودهن بنفسج يذوب الشحم والشمع ثم
يبرد ويجعل في الهاون ويذر عليه الكثيرا المسحوق
مثل الكحل وشيا من نشا مسحوق ويخلط معها ويستعمل
الباب الرابع عشر
في وجع الاسنان واللثه والضرس ينبغي ان يستقصي
موضع الوجع فان كان في اللثات فانها تلون وادمه
حمرا ويلون مع ذلك دلايل الدم ظاهره فالعلاج
الحجامه على النقره فان كنت والافصد القيفال والمضمض
بنقيع السماق والكسفره اليابسه او بما الفرع ويجعل
الغذا مبردا وان كان الوجع في اصول الاسنان ولاثان
صحيحه وعلامات الامتلا ظاهره نظر فان كان الامتلا
دمويا او صفراويا فصد العرق ثم سقي طبيخ الاهليلج
الاصفر والخيارشنبر وان كان الامتلا بلغميا او
سوداويا

٧٢

سودا او باسقي الايارج المركب اوحب الابلوج اوحب
القوقايي اوحب الاصطمخيقون وان لم ينق الامتلا
ظاهرا تمضمض العليل بخل قد طبخ فيه شي من قشور الحنظل
وشي من العاقرقرحا مرات كثيرة ولطف الغذا
واحد فيه مرات دهن المصطكي سخنا وان كان مع
السن تاكله حشيت بالقلونية الروميه اوحلتيت
او مصطكي وشي من قشور الافيون واما الضرس
فعلاجه العض على مح البيض المشوي الحار ومسح
الاسنان بالدهن المسخن واكل اللحم السمين الحار

الباب الخامس عشر

في بثور الفم والاسنان لحماة بالقلاع اذا كانت البثور
حمرا فالعلاج الحجامة على النقرة والمضمضة ورب
التوت ورب الحصرم ورب الريباس ومضغ اطراف
الكرم واللوز الرطب بقشره واكل الحلوا والزبيب
بدهن اللوز والسكر والحسا الشعير والتمر واكل

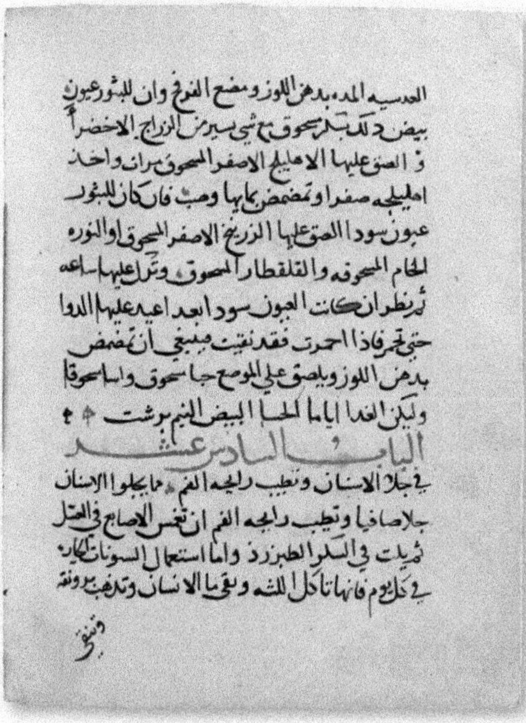

العدسيه المده بدهن اللوز ومضغ الفوخ وان للبثور عيون
بيض دلك بتكر سحوق مع شي يسير من الزاج الاخضر ثم
الصق عليها الاهليلج الاصفر المسحوق مرات واخذ
اهليلجه صفرا وتمضمض بمايها وصب فان كان للبثور
عيون سودا الصق عليها الزرنيخ الاصفر المسحوق او النوره
الحام المحرقه والقلقطار المحروق وترك عليها ساعه
ثم نظر ان كانت العيون سودا بعد اعيد عليها الدوا
حتى تحمر فاذا احمرت فقد نقيت فينبغي ان تمضمض
بدهن اللوز ويلصق علي الموضع جا سحوق واسا سحوقا
وليكن الغدا ايا ما لحسا البيض النيم برشت

الباب السادس عشر

في جلا الاسنان وتطيب رايحه الفم ❁ مما يجلوا الاسنان
جلا صافيا وتطيب رايحه الفم ان تغمس الاصابع في العسل
ثم يذر في السكر الطبرزد واما استعمال السونات الحاره
في كل يوم فانها تاكل اللثه وتعري الاسنان وتذهب برونقه

وتنقى

وتنفي رطوبه الفم فاما تطيب النكهه فينبغي ان يستعمل في
كل يوم اسبوع التمضمض بالسكنجبين المخلوط به شي من الملح
المسحوق تمضمضا مستقصي فان ذلك كاف لافراط
في استعماله

الباب التاسع عشر

في ورم اللهاه واللوزتين والخناق اذا ورمت
اللهاه واللوزتين وهما اصل الاذان في جانبي الحلق او
ورمت العضلات الداخله من الحلق او العضلات المطبقه
براس الحلقوم وراس المري فضاق النفس واشتد الامتداد
وكانت علامه الحراره ظاهره والبدن ممتليا فابدا بفصد
احد عروق المرفق ثم غرغر العليل الى اليوم الثالث بعصير
الرمان المدقوق بشحمه وبقشره وبرب الجوز الساذج
او بطبيخ الجلنار والورد والسماق واغذ العليل بما
الشعير الممزوج بما الرمان المز وان كان بعد البلال
فاسهل الطبيعه وان كان يجري الحلق بنفخ فبطبيخ الخيار
شنبر وغرغره بما التين وبلعاب بزر قطونا وبزر المرو

الابيض مع الناشيذ وغذه بصفرة البيض النيمبرشت
فان لم ينفع الحلق ولم يلن الازدراد فاحقنه بما الفاكهة
وطبيخ الحلبة والسكر الاحمر وان كان من البلغم والرطوبة
والحلب فلا تخرج الدم وغرغره برب الجوز الرطب
وان كان مجرى الحلق منفتحا فاسهله بطبيخ الخيار شنبر
والهليلج الاصفر والاسود فان لم يكن منفتحا فاحقنه
بحقنة قوية وحسه ما الحاله فاذا كان يوم الثلاث
فغرغره بما التين واصل السوس وان انفجر الورم وسال
القيح فاسقه ما العسل والجلاب الساذج او ما العسل الساذج
واذا انقطعت فانفخ في حلقه

الباب الثامن عشر

في العلق الناشب في الحلق اذا انشب العلق في الحلق
فانظر فان كان البصر يدركه فاجذبه بالكلبتين وان
كان غائبا عن البصر فجرع العليل نقيع الافسنتين فان
ذلك يقتلها ويجرع ما الترمس او ما الترمس المر ا
ويجرع العليل الخل الثقيف حارا تمت المقالة الرابعة

المقالة

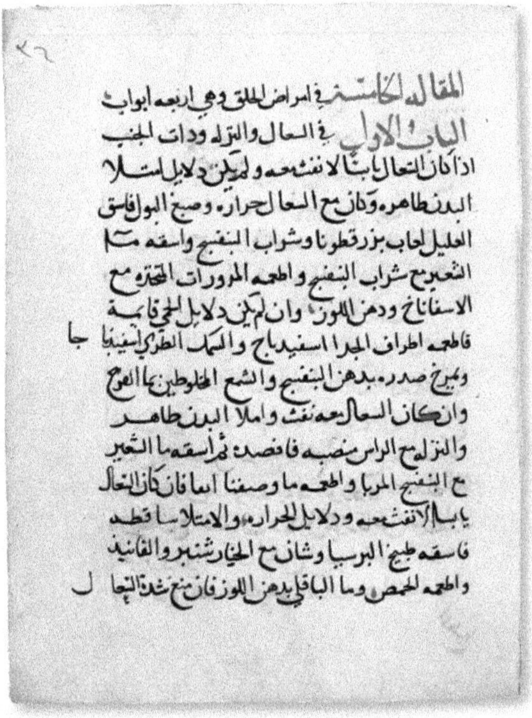

٤٦

المقالة الخامسة في امراض الحلق وهي اربعة ابواب

الباب الاول في السعال والنزلة وذات الجنب

اذا كان السعال يابسا لا نفث معه ولم يكن دلايل استلا

البدن ظاهره وكان مع السعال حرارة وصبغ البول فاسق

العليل لعاب بزرقطونا وشراب البنفسج واسقه ما

الشعير مع شراب البنفسج واطعمه المزورات المتخذة مع

الاسفاناخ ودهن اللوز وان لم يكن دلايل الحمى قايمة

فاطعمه اطراف الجدا اسفيدباج والسمك الطري اسفيدبا جا

ويمرخ صدره بدهن البنفسج والشمع المخلوطين بما القرع

وان كان السعال معه نفث وامتلا البدن ظاهر

والنزلة مع الراس منصبه فافصده ثم اسقه ما الشعير

مع البنفسج المربا واطعمه ما وصفنا انفا فان كان السعال

يابسا لا نفث معه ودلايل الحرارة والامتلا ساقطه

فاسقه طبيخ البرسيا وشان مع الخيارشنبر والفانيذ

واطعمه الحمص وما الباقلي بدهن اللوز فان منع شدة السعا ل

من النوم فاسقه شراب الخشخاش الساذج الباب الثاني
في الربو • إذا كان الانسان يصيبه النهز من المشي والحركات
العنيفة مع ضيق النفس وثقل الصدر فاسقه طبيخ
الزوفا واسقه لعوق العنصل بجوز مرو والتين الاصفر
واللوز المقشر مع العسل واطعمه ما الحمص بدهن الجوز
والشبث والكروبا اسقه الما الحار الذي قد لجيد عليه

الباب الثالث في الخفقان

اذا كان الخفقان مع امتلا البدن وعظم النبض فافصد
الباسليق الايسر واسق العليل اقراص الكافور برب التفاح
الساذج فاذا سكنت الحرارة فاسقه في كل يوم الاهليلج
المربا مع السكنجبين الساذج واطعمه الفروج بالحصرم
وبرده بخرق مصبوغة في ما الورد والصندل والكافور
فان كان مع الخفقان دلايل البرد فاسق العليل جوارشن
العنبر او دوا المسك للحلوم المنبه وشرب السوسن
فان كان مع ذلك فاسقه دوا المسك وحب الشبيار واسقه

المطبوخ

٢٧

المطبوخ العتيق وامرخ صدره بدهن السوسن والشمع
الاصفر وشمه الطيب ونخره. واطعمه الفراخ والعصا فير
زيرباجا فان كان الخفقان بعقب مرض واستفراغ
قوي فدبر العليل بالغذا المولد للدم واسقه الشراب
واسعه من الجماع

الباب الرابع

في نفث الدم متي خرج بالسعال دم فان كان الدم زبد
علي لون الورد فاسقه اقراص الكهربا الفرج ومتي كان
الدم احمر اسعا ولم تكن زبديا فاسق العليل اقراص
الكهربا واقراص الجلنار بما لسان الحمل وبما الرسايس
وطين المختوم مع الطباشير والورد والجلنار وبزر لسان
الحمل واسقه ما الحصرم والخل الممزوج وضمد الصدر
بالكندر ودم الاخوين والاقاقيا ودهن الورد والشمع
واطعمه المزورات المتخذه من العدس وما الحصرم وما
السماق والزيت الانفاق او دهن اللوز والنفل بالطين
الارمني والطباشير تمت المقاله الخامسة

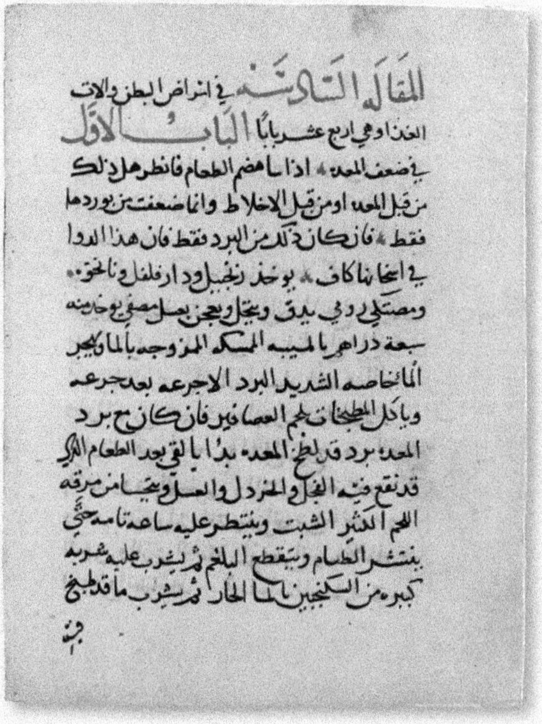

المقالة السادسة في امراض البطن والات
الغذا وهي اربع عشر بابا الباب الاول
في ضعف المعده اذا ساء هضم الطعام فانظر هل ذلك
من قبل المعده او من قبل الاخلاط وانما ضعفت من بوردها
فقط فان كان ذلك من البرد فقط فان هذا الدوا
في امحانا كاف يوخذ زنجبيل ودارفلفل ونانخوه
ومصطكي ودي بيدق ويحل ويعجن بعسل مصفى يوخذ منه
سبعة دراهم بالميبه المسكه الممزوجه بالما ويجير
الما خاصه الشديد البرد الا جرعه بعد جرعه
وياكل المطجنات لحم العصافير فان كان مع برد
المعده برد قد لطخ المعده بدا بالقي بعد الطعام الكثير
قد نقع فيه الفجل والخردل والعسل ويحسا من مرقه
اللحم الكثير الشبت وينتظر عليه ساعه تامه حتى
ينتشر الطعام ويتقطع البلغم ثم يشرب عليه شربه
كبيره من السكنجبين بالما الحار ثم يشرب ما قد طبخ
فيه

37B

٢٨

فيه اللوبيا الاحمر والملح الابيض والشبث ويقطر عليه
شيا من دهن الخل ثم يتقيا حتى يستنضف كلما اكل فاذا
نقي المعده اخذ المعجون الذي وصفنا . فانه كاف ان شا الله
فان كره القي او عسر عليه فاسقه كل ليله مثقالا من
حب الشبث الى ان تنقي معدته

الباب الثاني في الغثا .

اذا عرض الغثا بعد الاكل
فالعلاج في الطعام الماكول ثم شرب الماء واذا عرض
الغثا قبل الاكل فان كانت علامات الصفرا ظاهره
شرب ما باردا وحقا عا مبرد او يتكلف القي لتخرج الصفرا
المنصبه الى فم المعده ثم شرب ما الرمان الساذج وان
لم يكن علامات الصفرا ظاهره شرب ما الرمان
المتخذ بالنعناع فهو كاف في ذلك

الباب الثالث في المغص

متى حدث المغص بعقب الاكل فالعلاج القي
وخاصه ان كان الوجع في المعده فان كان الوجع
في السره مرخت السره بدهن الزنبق المسخن مع شي الملح

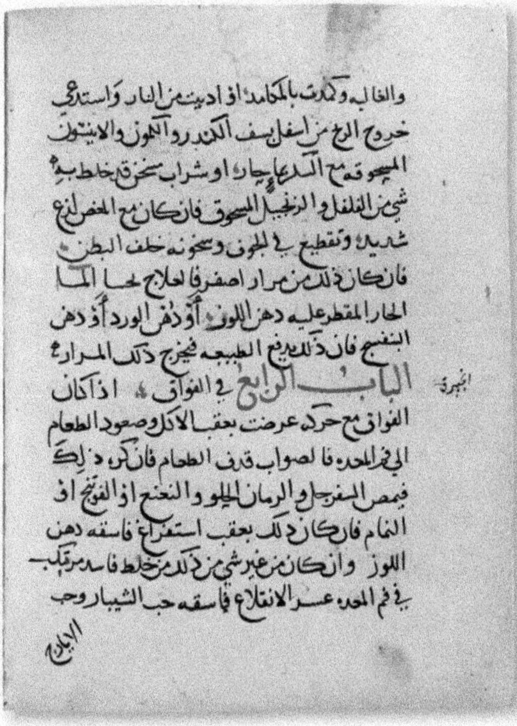
والغالبه وكمدت بالمكامد او اديت من النار واستدعي
خروج الريح من اسفل يسف الكندر والكمون والانيسون
المسحوقه مع السكر بماء حار او شراب سحق خلط به
شي من الفلفل والزنجبيل المسحوق فان كان مع المغص لذع
شديد وتقطيع في الجوف وسخونه خلف البطن
فان كان ذلك من مرار اصفر فالعلاج بحسا الماء
الحار المقطر عليه دهن اللوز او دهن الورد او دهن
البنفسج فان ذلك يدفع الطبيعه فيخرج ذلك المرار

الباب الرابع في الفواق اذا كان

الجبرى

الفواق مع حركه عرضت بعقب الاكل وصعود الطعام
الي فم المعده فالصواب قذف الطعام فان كره ذلك
فيمص السفرجل والرمان الحلو والنعنع او الفودنج او
النمام فان كان ذلك بعقب استفراغ فاسقه دهن
اللوز وان كان من غير شي من ذلك من خلط فاسد مرتكب
في فم المعده عسر الانقلاع فاسقه حب الشبيار وحب

الايارج

٢٤ زلاماج

ثم الطف الغذا او اسقه السكنجبين المحدث وقوفا المعده
بالاهليلج الكابلي ومما يسكن الفواق الحنيف ان يرد على الانسان
خبر عجيب فجاه حتى يشغل فكره ومنه ان يحبس الانسان نفسه
ويمدّ بانفه ساعه حتى يرجع نفسه الى جوفه

الباب الخامس في الهيضه

ان الهيضه تحدث اذا افرط مقدار الطعام فاذا ابتدات
المعده تهضمه عملت فيه عملا بقدر قوتها ثم تكل عن
تمام العمل فيبقى الطعام في حال سببه بنصف الانهضام
فتدفعه الطبع وكثيرا ما ينفتح المجاري وافواه العروق
المتصله بقعر المعده والامعا فيجلب اليها المرار في
البلغم فتصير الهيضه اسهالا فينبغي لمن تصيبه الهيضه
ان يتقيا ويخرج ما دام يخرج عنه غير منهضم وكان البدن
خفيف على ذلك القوه فينبغي الا يقطعه بل يستنظفه عن
آخره ويمسك عن الغذا يومه فان لم يقدر واخذ شيئا
من الخبز بمطبوخ عتيق فان كره المطبوخ فالمسه فاذا اشتد

البطن وهذا الوجع ووجد الوجع الصادق راجع الغذا
وخففه اياما فاذا افرط الاسهال وكان ما يخرج
مختلف اللون ولم يكن معه تقطيع ولا وجع وكان العهد
بشرب الدوا المسهل بعيدا فينبغي الا يحبس ما دامت
القوه لا تحور منه فان البدن ينقي به فاذا احدث معه
تقطيع ووجع وبدات القوه تسقط نظر فان كان ما
يخرج صفرا محض وكان العطش غالبا ولم يكن في البطن
قراقر ولا رياح فقد يكفي في حبس ذلك مخيض البقر مع
الكعك المحروق واذا احتيج الى دوا اخر وزن بزر
قطونا محمص يداف بما السماق المنقوع بالما ورد المصفى
ويشرب فان اشتد اللذع والتقطيع حقن بصفرة البيض
الحار مضروب بدهن الورد فان راي ان الانهاك
قد جرد المعا حقن بمرقة السكباج البقري بلب
الخبز وشرب عليه الما البارد وان كان ما يخرج
رطوبات وكان معه قراقر ورياح ولم يكن مع ذلك
عطش

عطش ولا لهيب اخذ وزن درهمين من الثوم المحرق
و وزن نصف درهم مصطكي ويداف برب الاس ويشرب
ويوكل عليه الباذروج بالزبيب الاسود و دهن الجوز
والريت ورعوه الخردل ويمزج ماه الخد يحون فان امسكت
الطبيعه عاود الغذا وجعله اياما مما يحبس البطن
فان كان مع الاسهال دم يسقى هذا الدوا يوخذ شي
من لسان الحمل وبزر الفرفخ وقلي ويسحق من كل واحد منهما
درهمين ومن الطين المختوم والصمغ العربي المقلو والطبا شير
من كل واحد درهم ويسف في مره واحده ويشرب
عليه شيا من عصير لسان الحمل وعصير الفرفخ ويجعل
غذاوه الكعك العتيق بالحصرم اوبما الرمان الحامض
او نقيع حب الرمان الحامض **الباب السادس**
في الزحير اذا ازعج الانسان البطن ازعاجا
متواترا وكان ما يخرج رطوبه بلغميه ذات رغوه
قليله المقدار فذلك هو الزحير وربما شاب ذلك

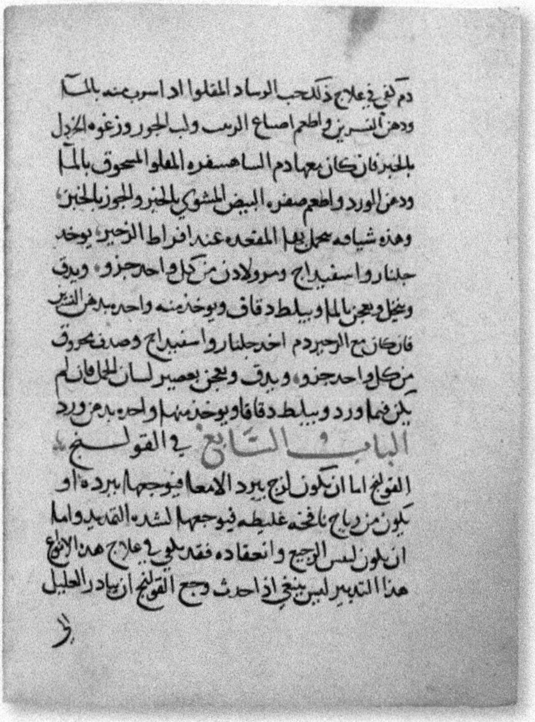
دم ثم في علاج ذلك حب الرساد المقلو اذا اسرب منه بالماء
ودهن النسرين واطعم اصابع الزينب ولب الجوز وزغوه الخردل
بالخبز فان كان معها دم الساهسفره المقلو المسحوق بالماء
ودهن الورد واطعم صفره البيض المشوي بالخبز والجوز بالخبز
وهذه شيافه تحمل بها المقعده عند افراط الزحير يوخذ
جلنار واسفيداج وسرولادن من كل واحد جزو ويدق
وينخل ويعجن بالماء ويبلط دقاق ويوخذ منه واحد بدهن النسرين
فان كان مع الزحير دم اخذ جلنار واسفيداج وصدف محروق
من كل واحد جزو ويدق ويعجن بعصير لسان الحمل فان لم
يكن فماء ورد ويبلط دقاقا ويوخذ منها واحد بدهن ورد
الباب التاسع في القولنج
القولنج اما ان يكون لزج يبرد الامعا فيوجعها ببرده او
يكون من رياح نافخه غليظه فيوجعها لشده التمديد واما
ان يكون لبس الرجيع وانعقاده فقد يلي في علاج هذه الانواع
هذا التدبير لبين ينبغي اذا احدث وجع القولنج ان يبادر العليل
ان

٤١

الي شرب الادويه الحاره ولا المسهله خاصة ان كان قريب
العهد بالطعام فان ذلك يزيد في الوجع ويقوي العله ويجلب
افات كثيره لكن ينبغي ان يمسك عن الطعام ويتجرع الما الشديد
الحراره جرعه جرعه حتي تنقضي سوره العله وتسكن حميه
الوجع وحد الامساك عن الطعام اقله يومان فان كان العليل
خوار الجوع من ترك الغذا احسي شيا من ما اللحم المحدد بالتوابل
بشي يسير من لب الخبز ثم يسقي من الايارج الفيقرا المعجون السادج
درهمين وانتظر عليه اربع ساعات ثم اتبعه بهذا المطبوخ وهو
ان يوخذ قشور اصل الكرفس وقشور اصل الرازيانج من كل واحد
وزن عشره دراهم بزر الكرفس وبزر الرازيانج وكمون من كل
واحد وزن درهمين يطبخ ذلك علي ثلثه ارطال ما حتي يرجع الي
رطل واحد ويصفي منه ثلثا رطل ويمرس فيه من فلوس الخيار
شنبر وزن سبعه دراهم ومن الغاريقون وزن ثلثه دراهم
ويشرب حارا فان كانت دلايل الحراره ظاهره او كان
العليل محرورا جعل بدل دهن الخروع وزن درهم ونصف

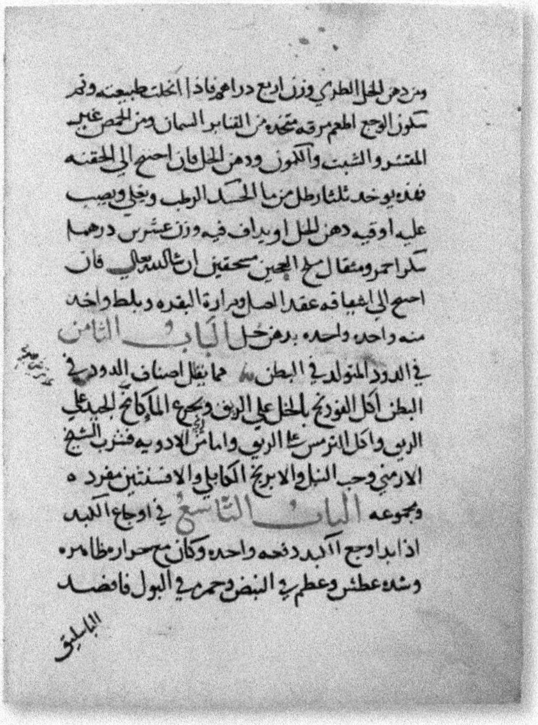

ومن دهن الخل الطري وزن اربع دراهم فاذا انحلت طبيعته وتم
سكون الوجع اطعم مرقه متخذه من القنابر السمان ومن الحمص غير
المقشر والشبت والكمون ودهن الخل فان احتيج الي الحقنه
فقد يوخذ ثلث رطل من ما الحسك الرطب ويغلي ويصب
عليه اوقيه دهن الخل او يداف فيه وزن عشرين درهما
سكر احمر ومثقال ملح الهجين سحقين ان شا الله تعالي فان
احتيج الي الشيافه عقد الصل ومرارة البقره ويلط واخذ
منه واحده واحده بدهن خل الباب الثامن
في الدود المتولد في البطن مما يقتل اصناف الدود في
البطن اكل الفودنج بالخل علي الريق وشرب الماء كامخ الحيتكي علي
الريق واكل الترمس علي الريق واما من الادويه فشرب الشيح
الارمني وحب النيل والابرنج الكابلي والافسنتين مفرد ه
ومجموعه الباب التاسع في اوجاع الكبد
اذا ابدا وجع الكبد دفعه واحده وكان مع حرارة ظاهره
وشده عطش وعظم في النبض وحمره في البول فافصد
الباسليق

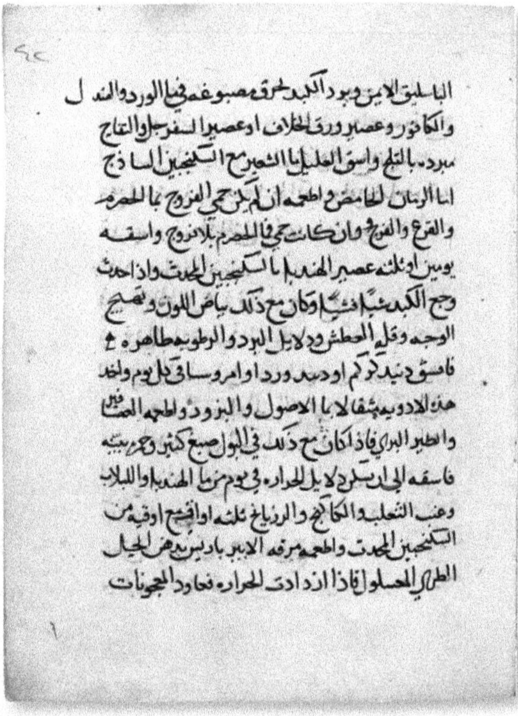

البا سليق الايمن ويبرد الكبد بخرقة مصبوغة في ماء الورد والصندل
والكافور وعصير ورق الخلاف او عصير السفرجل او التفاح
مبرد بالثلج واسق العليل ماء الشعير مع السكنجبين الساذج
او ماء الرمان الحامض واطعمه ان لم يكن حمى المزوج بماء الحصرم
والقرع والفروج وان كانت حمى فالحصرم بلا فروج واسقه
يومين او ثلثة عصير الهندبا بالسكنجبين المحدث واذا احدث
وجع الكبد شيئا فشيئا وكان مع ذلك بياض اللون وتهيج
الوجه وقلة العطش ودلائل البرد والرطوبة ظاهرة
فاسق دينار كوكم او دستة ورد او امروساني كل يوم ولتكن
هذه الادوية مطبوخة بماء الاصول والبزور واطعمه العصافير
والطير البري فاذا كان مع ذلك في البول صبغ كثير وحرقة
فاسقه الجلاب بعد دلائل الحرارة في يوم من ماء الهندبا واللبلاب
وعنب الثعلب والكاكنج والرازيانج ثلثة اواق مع اوقية من
السكنجبين المحدث واطعمه مرقة الاسفيدباج بدهن الجبل
الطري المغسول فاذا ازدادت الحرارة فعاود المعجونات

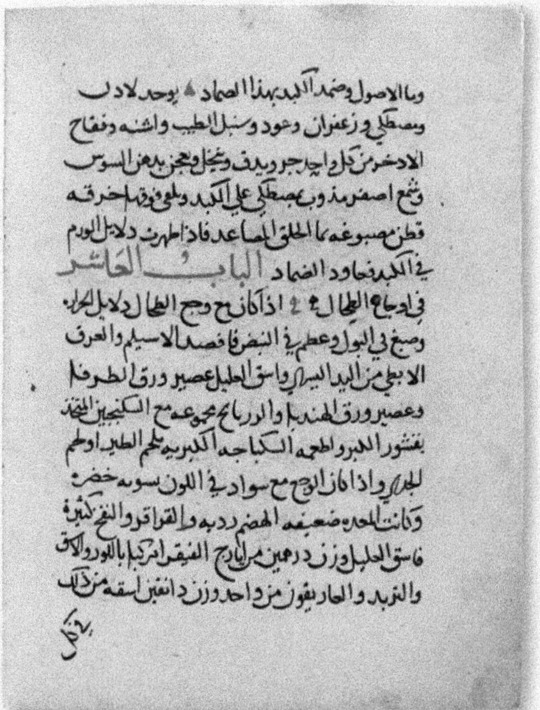

وما الاصول وضمد الكبد بهذا الضماد ◆ يوخذ لادن
ومصطكي وزعفران وعود وسنبل الطيب واشنه وتفاح
الاذخر من كل واحد جزو ويدق وينخل ويعجن بدهن السوسن
وشمع اصفر مذوب ويصطكى على الكبد ويلقى فوقها خرقه
قطن مصبوغه بما الحلق الصاعد فاذا ظهرت دلايل الورم
في الكبد فجاوز الضماد الباب العاشر
في اوجاع الطحال ◆ اذا كان مع وجع الطحال دلايل الحراره
وصبغ في البول وعظم في النبض فافصد الاسيليم والعرق
الابطي من اليد اليسرى واسق العليل عصير ورق الطرفا
وعصير ورق الهندبا والريباس مجموعه مع السكنجبين المتخذ
بقشور الكبر واطعمه السكباجة الكبريه بلحم الطير او لحم
الجدي واذا كان الوجع مع سواد في اللون سوبه خضرة
وكانت المعده ضعيفه الهضم رديه والقراقر والنفخ كثيرة
فاسق العليل وزن درهمين من اياريج الفيقرا مركبا بالورد والك
والتربد والغاريقون من واحد وزن دانقين اسقه من ذلك
بعض

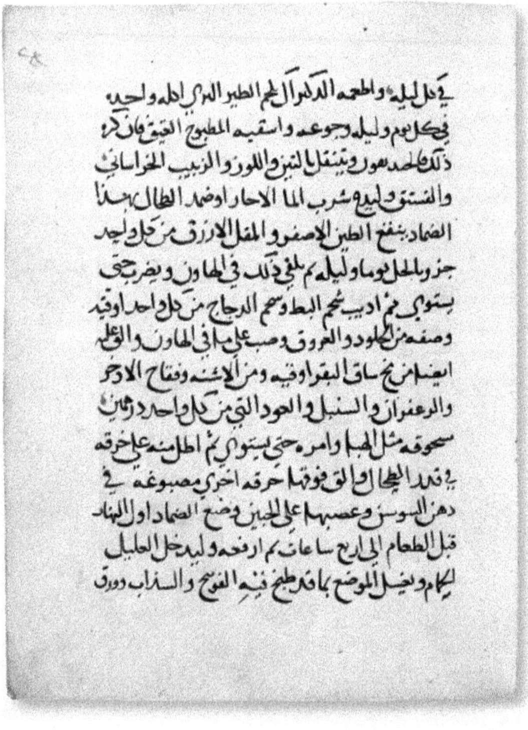
في كل ليلة واطعمه الدكر اكل لحم الطير البري اطله واحده
في كل يوم وليلة وجوعه واسقيه المطبوخ العتيق وان كره
ذلك الحد سور ويتنقل بالتين واللوز والزبيب الخراساني
والفستق وليدع شرب الما الاحار اوضمد الطحال بهذا
الضماد ينفع الطين الاصفر والمقل الازرق من كل واحد
جز وبالخل يوما وليله ثم يلقي ذلك في الهاون ويضرب حتى
يستوي ثم اذيب شحم البط وشحم الدجاج من كل واحد اوقيه
وصفه من الجلود والعروق وصب على ما في الهاون والق عليه
ايضا مخ ساق البقر اوقيه ومن الاشنه وتفاح الاذخر
والزعفران والسنبل والعود التي من كل واحد درهمين
مسحوقه مثل الهبا وامره حتى يستوي ثم اطل منه على خرقه
بقدر الطحال والق فوقها خرقه اخرى مصبوغه في
دهن السوسن وعصبها على الجبين وضع الضماد اول النهار
قبل الطعام الى اربع ساعات ثم ارفعه وليدخل العليل
الحمام وتغسل الموضع بما قد طبخ فيه القيصوم والسذاب دورق

الفنجنكشت وورق الطرفا الباب الحادي عشر
في اليرقان اذا اصفر جلد الجسد عامه والحدقتان
خاصه وكان مع ذلك حمى حاده فان اليرقان عند ذلك تابع
في اكثر الامر لسوء مزاج فان بعد ذلك يكون بحران الحمى والسلامه
منها وعلاج هذه الحمى علاج اليرقان سوا واذا حدث اليرقان
الصحيح الذي لا حمى به وكان مع ذلك دلايل الحراره فاسق
العليل ما الهندبا والرازيانج مع السكنجبين الحمض وليدخل العليل
ابزن الحمام في كل يوم قبل الطعام واسهل طبيعته بطبيخ الاهليلج
الاصفر والخيار شنبر والسكر الطبرزد فاذا لم يسق الاصفر
الحرقه فاسعط العليل بقطرات من الخل المضروب ودهن
الورد في كل يوم واطعمه السكباج بلحم الفروج الشديد
الحموضه والقريص والمصوص واذا لم يكن مع اليرقان
شي من دلايل الحراره وكان انما حدث بعقب ادمان الاطعمه
الغليظه اللزجه فاسق العليل حب الغافت في كل ليلة وزن
درهمين واسقه من اللحم ولطف غذاه واطعمه المزورات الحامضه

برهن

٤٢

بدهن الخل

الباب الثاني عشر

في امراض الكلتين اذا عرض في الكلتين وجع دفعه
واحده وكان ذلك عقيب ادمان اللحم والحلوا وشرب النبيذ
وكان مع ذلك في النبض عظم وفي البول حمره فافصد العليل البا سليق
من الجانب الوجع ولطف غذا العليل واطعمه المزورات
المتخذه من الاسفاناخ والقرع والمح المقشر ودهن اللوز والعدس
المقشر واسقه بالغداوت بزر البطيخ والخيار والقثا
والقرع مقشوره مع بزر الخشخاش الابيض والطباشير
بشراب البنفسج فان لم يكف ذلك فاطلق الطبيعه بما الفاكهه
بدهن الورد الخام المضروب مع ما الورد وان كان العليل
بعيد العهد بالجماع فليجامع فان حدث مع ذلك عطش شديد
مفرط فاسق العليل مع ذلك ما الشعير المطبوخ بالقرع
واسقه مخيض البقر بالكعك واطعمه السمك الطري سكباجا
والفروج بالحصرم واطعمه البطيخ السندي ولب الخيار
وسويق الشعير بالما المبرد بالثلج واطل على موضع الكليه

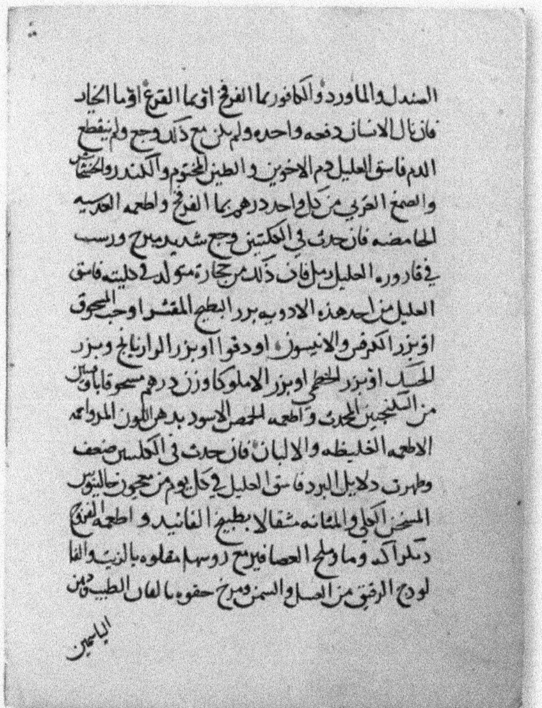
الصندل والماورد والكافور بما الفرخ اى بما القرع او ما الخيار
فان بال الانسان دفعه واحده ولم يكن مع ذلك وجع ولم ينقطع
الدم فاسق العليل دم الاخوين والطين المختوم والكندر والخشخاش
والصمغ العربي من كل واحد درهم بما الفرخ واطعمه العدسيه
الحامضه فان حدث في الكليتين وجع شديد مبرح ورسب
في قاروره العليل رمل فان ذلك من حجاره متولده في كليته فاسق
العليل من احد هذه الادويه بزر البطيخ المقشر او حب المحروق
او بزر الكرفس والانيسون او دقو او بزر الرازيانج وبزر
الحسك او بزر الخطمي او بزر الاملوكا وزن درهم مسحوقا باوقيه من
السكنجبين [illegible] واطعمه الحمص الاسود بدهن اللوز المر واحمه
الاطعمه الغليظه والالبان فان حدث في الكليتين ضعف
وظهرت دلايل البرد فاسق العليل في كل يوم من معجون جالينوس
المسخن للكلى والمثانه مثقالا بطبيخ الفانيد واطعمه الفروج
ولحم الديك وما ولحم العصافير مع روسهم مقلوه بالزيت والفا
لوذج الرقيق من العسل والسمن ومرخ حقوه بالعال الطيب ودهن
الياسمين

٤٩

الياسمين مع الغاليه واسقه الشراب وليبع ليلحام مده طويله

الباب الثالث عشر في امراض المثانه

اذا تولدت الحصاه في المثانه واكثر ذلك تكون في الصبيان
فيدل عليها البول الابيض والرمل الابيض الراسب فيه وسوسر
القضيب والحكه الدايمه فيه فاسق العليل من الحواي مرحبه
الى دانق على قدر القوه السن بطبيخ الناخوه والقاشيه واسقه
من بزر الكرفس الجبلي السحق من دانق الى نصف درهم بما العسل
واطعمه الحليه والجزر به بدهن الحل ودهن الجوز فاذا احدث
بالانسان تقطير البول فان كان البول اصفر حادا او دلايل
الحراره ظاهره فاسق العليل البزور البارده التي وصفنا
بشراب البنفسج واسقه المخيض بالكعك واطعمه مزوره الاسفاناخ ناخ
بدهن اللوز وان افرط حرقه البول فاسقه اللبن الحليب
بالسكر واعصر طبيخته بما الحسر المركب فاذا لم يكن مع تقطير
البول حرقه ولا لدع وكان البول ابيض والبرد والرطوبه
ظاهرين فاسق العليل البحريا فيحون حالينوس والبوب الحاره

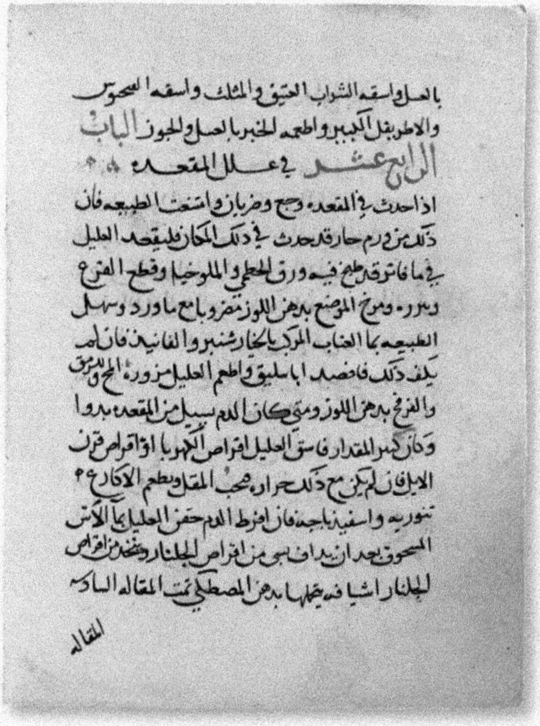

بالعسل واسقه الشراب العتيق والمثلث واسقه المحروس
والاطريفل الكبير واطعمه الخبز بالعسل والجوز الباب
الرابع عشر في علل المقعدة

اذا احدث في المقعدة وجع وضربان واشتغلت الطبيعة فان
ذلك من ورم حار قد حدث في ذلك المكان فليقعد العليل
في ما فاتر قد طبخ فيه ورق الخطمي والملوخيا وقطع القرع
وبزره ومرخ الموضع بدهن اللوز مضروبا مع ماورد وسهل
الطبيعة بما العناب المركب بالخيارشنبر والفانيذ فان لم
يكف ذلك فافصد الباسليق واطعم العليل مزورة الجح والدرمق
والفرخ بدهن اللوز ومتى كان الدم يسيل من المقعدة بدوا
وكان كثير المقدار فاسق العليل اقراص الكهربا او اقراص قرن
الايل ان لم يكن مع ذلك حرارة صحبت المقل وبطعم الاكارع
تنوريه واسفيذباجة فان افرط الدم حقن العليل بما الاس
المسحوق بعد ان يذاف بشي من اقراص الجلنار وتتخذ من اقراص
الجلنار اشيافا فيحملها بدهن المصطكي تمت المقالة السادسة

المقالة

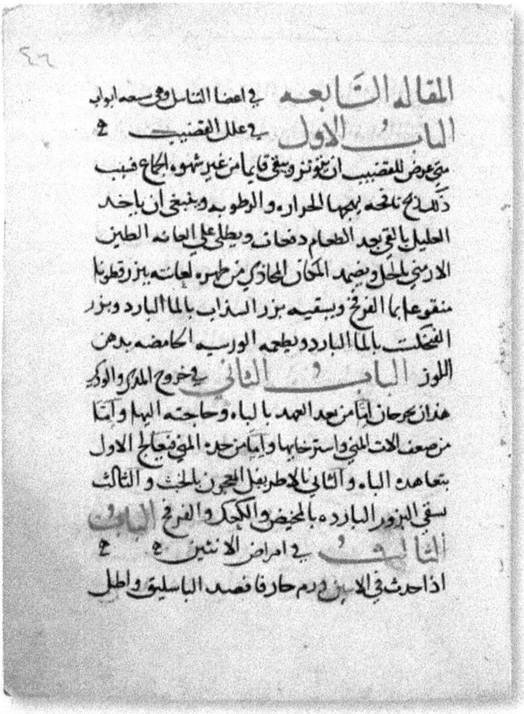

٤٦

المقالة الرابعة في اعضا التناسل وهي سبعة ابواب
الباب الاول في علل القضيب ح
متى عرض للقضيب ان يتوتر ويبقى قايما من غير شهوة الجماع فسبب
ذلك ريح نافخة سببها الحرارة والرطوبة وينبغي ان ياخذ
العليل بالقي بعد الطعام دفعات ويطلى على العانة الطين
الارمني بالخل ويضمد المكان المحاذي من ظهره لعانته ببزر قطونا
منقوعا بما الفرفخ ويسقيه بزر السذاب بالما البارد وبزر
الفنجنكشت بالما البارد ويطعمه الورسيه الحامضه بدهن
اللوز الباب الثاني في خروج المذي والودي
هذان يعرضان اما من بعد العهد بالباه وحاجته اليها واما
من ضعف الات المني واسترخايها واما من حدة المني فيعالج الاول
بتعاهد الباه والثاني بالاطريفل المعجون بالخبث والثالث
سقي البزور البارده بالمخيض والكعك والفرفخ الباب
الثالث في امراض الانثيين ح ح
اذا حدث في الانثيين ورم حار فافصد الباسليق واطل

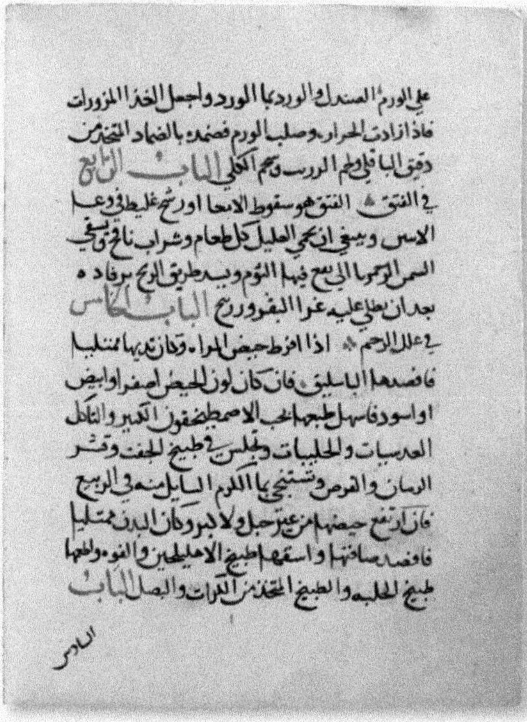
علي الورم الصندل والورد بما الورد والجمل الخدا المزورات
فاذا ازادت الحرارة وصلب الورم فضمده بالضماد المتخذ من
دقيق الباقلي ولحم الزبيب وبحم الكلي الباب الرابع
في الفتق ❁ الفتق هو سقوط الامعا او ثرب غليظ في وعا
الاسس وينبغي ان يحمي العليل كل طعام وشراب نافخ وينبغي
السمن الزيتيا التي يقع فيها النوم ويشد طريق الريح برفاده
بعد ان يطلي عليه غرا البقر ورد الباب الخامس
في علل الرحم ❁ اذا افرط حيض المراة وكان بدنها ممتليا
فافصدها الباسليق فان كان لون الحيض اصفر او ابيض
او اسود فاسهل طبعها بحب الاصطمخيقون الكبير والتاكل
العدسيات والحلبيات وتجلس في طبيخ الجفت وقشر
الرمان والعفص وتستنجي بما اللحم السايل منه في الربيع
فان ارتفع حيضها من غير حبل ولا كبر وكان البدن ممتليا
فافصد صافنها واسقها طبيخ الاهليلجين والفوه والجعدة
طبيخ الحلبة والطبيخ المتخذ من الكراث والبصل الباب
السادس

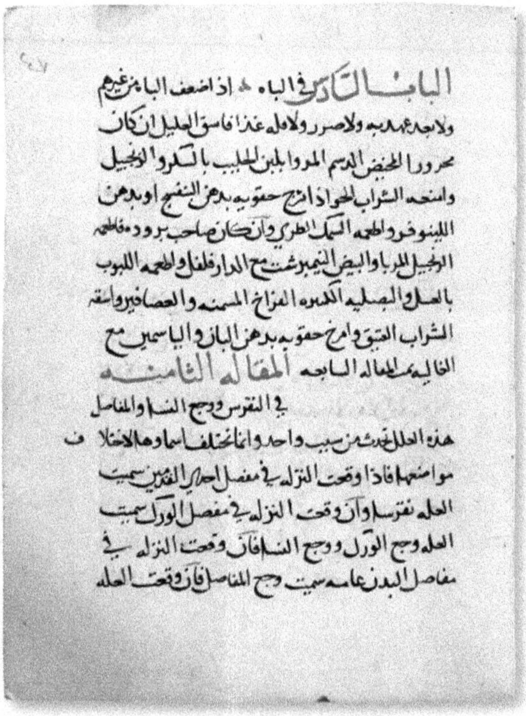

الباب السادس في الباه اذا ضعف الباه من غيرهم
ولا بعد عهد به ولا اصرر ولا قلة غذا فاسق العليل ان كان
محرورا الحنيض الدسم المزوا بلبن الحليب بالسكر والنجيل
واسقه الشراب الحلو واذا مزج حقويه بدهن البنفسج او بدهن
اللينوفر واطعمه السمك الطري وان كان صاحب برودة فاطعمه
الزنجبيل المربا والبيض النيمبرشت مع الدار فلفل واطعمه اللبوب
بالعسل والبصليه الكمبوه الفراخ المسمنه والعصافير واسقه
الشراب العتيق وامرخ حقويه بدهن البان والياسمين مع
الغاليه تمت المقالة السابعه المقالة الثامنه

في النقرس ووجع النسا والمفاصل

هذه العلل تحدث من سبب واحد وانما تختلف اسماوها لاختلاف
مواضعها فاذا وقعت النزلة في مفصل احد القدمين سميت
العله نقرسا وان وقعت النزلة في مفصل الورك سميت
العله وجع الورك ووجع النسا فان وقعت النزلة في
مفاصل البدن عامه سميت وجع المفاصل فان وقعت العله

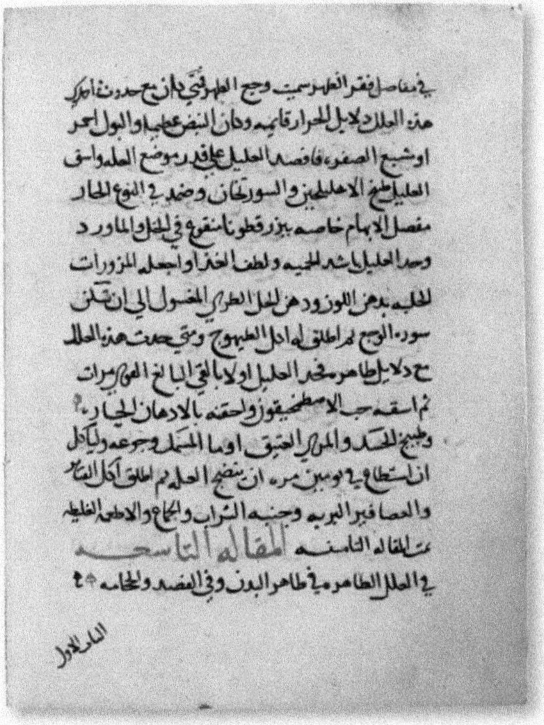
في مفاصل فقر الظهر سميت وجع الظهر فمتى دان مع حدوث احد
هذه العلل دلايل الحرارة قايمه وكان النبض عظيما والبول احمر
او شبيع الصفرة فافصد العليل على قدر موضع العله واسق
العليل طبيخ الاهليلجين والسورنجان وضمد في النوع الحار
مفصل الابهام خاصه ببزر قطونا منقوع في الخل والماورد
وسد العليل باشد الحميه ولطف الغذا واجعله المزورات
المطبوخه بدهن اللوز ودهن الخل الطري المغسول الى ان تسكن
سورة الوجع ثم اطلق له اكل الطيهوج ومتى حدثت هذه العلل
مع دلايل ظاهره فخذ العليل اولا بالقي البالغ القوي مرات
ثم اسقه حب الاصطمخيقون واحقنه بالادهان الحاره
وطبيخ الحسك والمري العتيق او ماء المسلح وجرعه ولياكل
ان استطاع في يومين مره ان نضج العله ثم اطلق اكل العصافير
والعصافير البريه وجنبه الشراب والجماع والاطعمة الغليظه
تمت المقاله الثامنه المقاله التاسعه
في العلل الظاهره في ظاهر البدن وفي الفصد والحجامه

٤٨

الباب الاول في تمرط الشعر

اذا انمرط شعر اللحيه والراس والاشفار فالزم العليل الحمية
تنقي معدته ثم انظر فان كان البدن ممتليا والنبض عظيما والبو ل
احمرا واصفر مشبعا فافصده ثم الزمه حب الايارج الي
ان يبرا واطعمه الخبز النقي الابيض وجنبه الالبان والتمور
والمالح والخريف كله والباه فان لم تكن علامات الدم ظاهره
فدع الفصد واجر سائر التدبير علي ما وصفنا فاما الحزاز
وتشقق الشعر فاذا غلب فعلاجه تنقيه البدن والراس
بما وصفنا فاذا اجتمع فيه الحلق ان كان في الراس وغسل
بالخطمي والبورق وورق الاهليلج وحماية استاصل الحزاز ادمان
الاستعاط بالدهن في كل ليله الا ان يمنع مانع

الباب الثاني في جلا الوجه من الكلف والنمش

متي كان هذا غليظ بدي في علاجه بفصد العروق فان
كان البدن ممتليا فيسقي طبيخ الافيثمون والغاريقون ثم
يطلي علي الموضع بزر الجرجير حتي يقرح الجلد وياكل الفساد

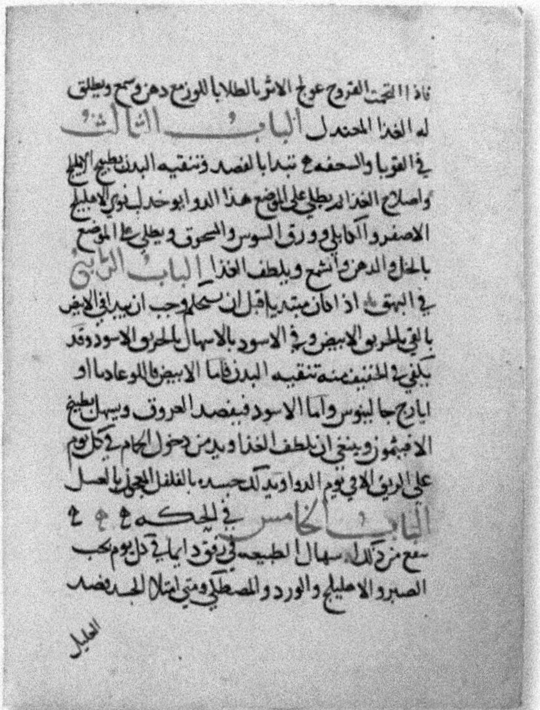

فاذا انفتحت القروح عولج الاثر بالطلا باللوز مع دهن وشمع ويطلق
له الغذا المعتدل الباب الثالث
في القوبا والسعفة تبدا بالفصد وتنقيه البدن بطبيخ الاهليلج
واصلاح الغذا ثم يطلي على الموضع هذا الدوا يوخذ لب نوى الاهليلج
الاصفر والكابلي وورق السوسن والمحرق ويطلي على الموضع
بالخل والدهن والشمع ويلطف الغذا الباب الرابع
في البهق اذا كان مبتديا قبل ان يستحكم وجب ان يبدا في الابيض
بالقي بالخربق الابيض وفي الاسود بالاسهال بالخربق الاسود وقد
يكفي في الخفيف منه تنقيه البدن فاما الابيض فاللوغاذيا او
ايارج جالينوس واما الاسود فيفصد العروق ويسهل بطبيخ
الافتيمون وينبغي ان يلطف الغذا ويدمن دخول الحمام في كل يوم
على الريق الا في يوم الدوا ويدلك جسده بالفلفل المعجون بالعسل
الباب الخامس في الحكة
ينفع من ذلك اسهال الطبيعة في زموره ايارج في كل يوم بحب
الصبر والاهليلج والورد والمصطكي ومتى امتلا الجسد فصد
العليل

٢٩

العلل ثم اعيد الي الاسهال بالرفق فاذا انقيت عروقه فليواظب
علي الحمام ويدلك جسده بالاشنان الاخضر حتي يبرا ويكون غذاوه
اللحم الخفيف والخبز النقي وينهي عن الشراب والباه

الباب الثاني في الجدري والحصبة والشري والحصف

علاج الجدري والحصبة الكائنين بعد ظهور الحمي والبثور سقيا ماء الشعير
والغذ بالعدس المقشور وسقي الجلاب او ماء الرمان [illegible] ودهن
الورد مضروبين وقطر الماورد في عينيه بطرف الميل فان
لانت الطبيعة سقي ماء سويق الشعير غذا با العدس بعد ان
يغلي ويسقي ربوب الفاكهة فاذا تفتحت البثور دخن بالطرفا
وزر ورد وينثر في فراشه الورد والاس المسحوقان فاذا
دخت الحمي واستمسكت الطبيعة اطلق له الفروج بماء الحصرم
او بماء الرمان فاما الشري فينبغي في علاجه القعود في
الما الجاري ويلطف الغذا فاذا دام وصعب عولج بالفصد
وسقي طبيخ الاهليلج واما الحصف فينبغي ان يعالج اذا ظهر فصب
الما البارد عليه ثم يمسحه بالماورد

الباب الثالث

[illegible]

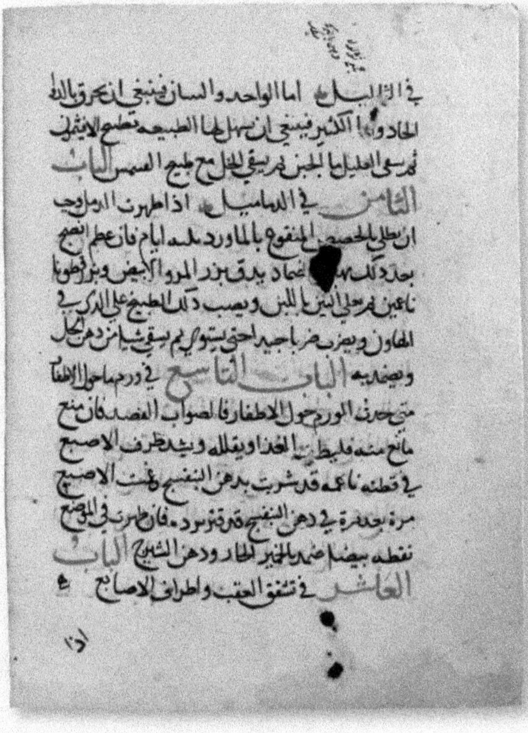

في الثآليل أما الواحد والاثنان فينبغي أن يحرق بالدواء
الحاد وأما الكثير فينبغي أن يسهل لها الطبيعة وتطلى الاثاليل
ثم يسحق العليل بالجبن ثم يبقى الخل مع طبيخ العدس الباب
الثامن في الدماميل إذا ظهرت الدماميل وجب
أن يطلى بالحمص المنقوع بالماورد ثلاثة أيام فإن عظم انضج
بعد ذلك بضماد يدق بزر المرو الأبيض وبزر قطونا
ناعمين ثم يطلى الشيرج باللبن ويصب ذلك الطبيخ على الدرك في
الهاون ويضرب ضربا جيدا حتى يستوي ثم يسقى شيئا من دهن الخل
ويضمد به الباب التاسع في ورم ما حول الاظفار
متى حدث الورم حول الاظفار فالصواب الفصد فإن منع
مانع منه فليطلى الغذاء ويقلله ويشد طرف الاصبع
في قطنة ناعمة قد شربت بدهن البنفسج ويغمس الاصبع
مرة بعد مرة في دهن البنفسج قد فتر برد فإن ظهرت في الموضع
نقطة بيضاء ضمد بالخبز الحار ودهن الشيرج الباب
العاشر في تشقق العقب وأطراف الأصابع

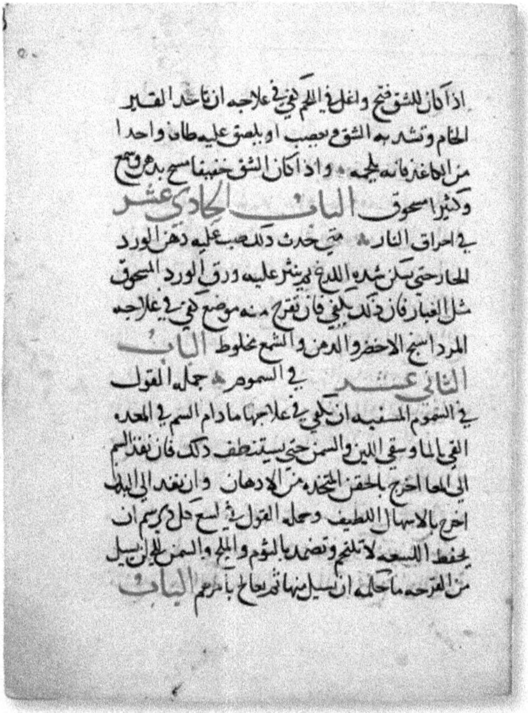

اذا كان للشق فتح واغلق في اللحم نفي في علاجه ان تاخذ القير
الحام وتشد به الشق وتعصب او يلصق عليه طاق واحد
من الكاغذ فانه يلحمه • واذا كان الشق خفيفا مسح بدهن وتمع
وكثيرا مسحوق الباب الحادي عشر
في احراق النار • متى حدث ذلك صب عليه دهن الورد
الحار حتى يسكن شدة اللدغ ثم ينثر عليه ورق الورد المسحوق
مثل الغبار فان ذلك يكفي فان تقرح منه موضع كفي في علاجه
المرداسنج الاخضر والدهن والشمع مخلوط الباب
الثاني عشر في السموم • جملة القول
في السموم المشروبة ان يكفي في علاجها ما دام السم في المعدة
القي بالماء وسقي اللبن والسمن حتى يستنظف ذلك فان نفذ السم
الى المعا اخرج بالحقن المتخذة من الادهان وان نفذ الى البدن
اخرج بالاسهال اللطيف وجملة القول في لسع كل دبيب ان
يحفظ اللسعة لا تلتحم وتضمد بالثوم والملح والسمن الى ان يسيل
من القرحة ما حاله ان يسيل منها ثم يعالج بالمرهم الباب

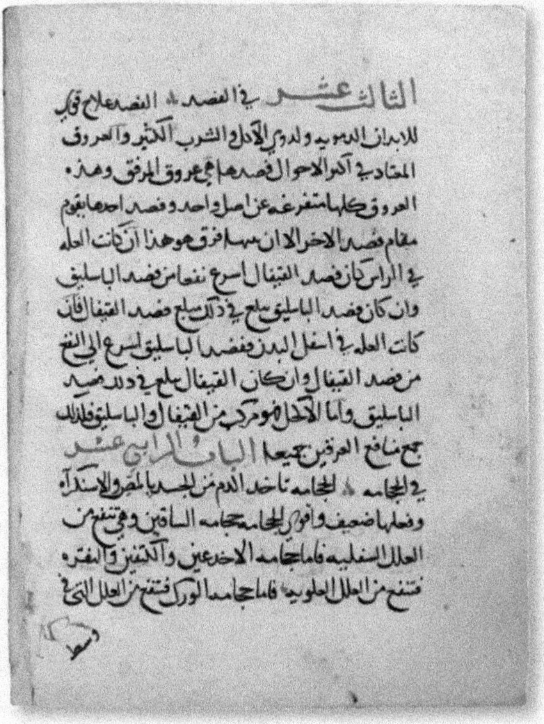

الثالث عشر في الفصد . الفصد علاج قوي
للابدان الدموية ولذوي الأكل والشرب الكثير والعروق
المعتاد في اكثر الاحوال فصدها هي عروق المرفق وهذه
العروق كلها متفرعة عن اصل واحد وفصد احدها يقوم
مقام فصد الاخر الا ان بينها فرق وهو هذا ان كانت العلة
في الراس كان فصد القيفال اسرع نفعا من فصد الباسليق
وان كان فصد الباسليق يبلغ في ذلك مبلغ فصد القيفال فان
كانت العلة في اسفل البدن ففصد الباسليق اسرع الى النفع
من فصد القيفال وان كان القيفال يبلغ في ذلك مبلغ
الباسليق واما الأكحل فهو مركب من القيفال والباسليق فلذلك
جمع منافع العرقين جميعا الباب الرابع عشر
في الحجامة . الحجامة تاخذ الدم من الجسد بالمص والاستدرار
وفعلها ضعيف وانفع الحجامة حجامة الساقين وهي تنفع من
العلل السفلية فاما حجامة الاخدعين والكتفين والنقرة
فتنفع من العلل العلوية فاما حجامة الورك فتنفع من العلل التي في

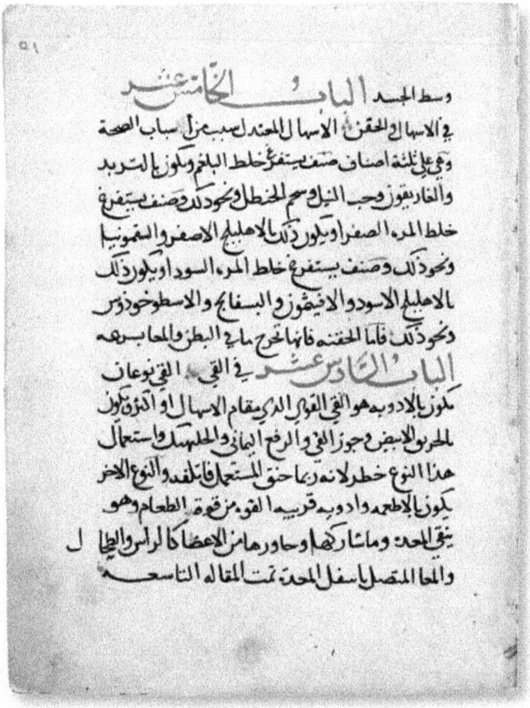

٥١

وسط الجسد الباب الخامس عشر

في الاسهال والحقنة الاسهال المعتدل سبب من اسباب الصحة
وهي على ثلثة اصناف صنف يستفرغ خلط البلغم ويكون بالتربد
والغاريقون وحب النيل وشحم الحنظل ونحو ذلك وصنف يستفرغ
خلط المرة الصفراء ويكون ذلك بالاهليلج الاصفر والسقمونيا
ونحو ذلك وصنف يستفرغ خلط المرة السوداء ويكون ذلك
بالاهليلج الاسود والافيثمون والبسفايج والاسطوخودوس
ونحو ذلك فاما الحقنة فانها تخرج ما في البطن والمعا برفقه

الباب السادس عشر في القي القي نوعان

يكون بالادوية هو القي القوي الذي يقام الاسهال او اكثر يكون
بالخربق الابيض وجوز القي والرفع اليماني والخلهنك واستعمال
هذا النوع خطر لانه ربما خنق المستعمل فاتلفه والنوع الاخر
يكون بالاطعمة والادوية قريبة القوة من قوة الطعام وهو
ينقي المعدة وما شاركها وجاورها من الاعضا كالراس والطحال ل
والمعا المتصل باسفل المعدة تمت المقالة التاسعة

المقالة العاشرة في الحميات وهي سبعة ابواب
الباب الاول في حمى يوم ۞ هذه الحمى تحدث من التعب
الشديد ومن التعرض للشمس الحارة والبرد الشديد ومن
الاغذية الحارة ومن الغضب الشديد والغم الشديد ولها
اسباب تتابعه لهذه الاسباب وهي تمكث اربعة وعشرين ساعة
ومتى عرضت هذه فينبغي ان ترفق بصاحبها ولا تحرك ... تنحل
حمي يانيه وان يطفيها بالاشربة والربوب بخز وجه بالما البارد
وان كان قريب العهد بالطعام وعلم ان ترك الاكل لا يزيد في حره
حماه اقتصرت على الاشربة والربوب الباردة فان خاف زيادة
الحمى اكل يسيرا من السويق المبرد مع شي من السكر اليسير وشي يسير
من الخبز المغسول بما الرمان المز واذا زالت الحمي دخل الحمام
وعاود الغذا برفق الباب الثاني
في الحمى التي تنوب في كل يوم وهي البلغم ۞ هذه الحمى تتولد من البلغم
العفن اذا غلب على المعدة وعروق البدن وينبغي في علاج هذه
اذا كانت خالصة ولم يكن صاحبها شرها سقيه المعدة بالقي

٥٢

بطبيخ الخل والسكنجبين العسلي واكل الخل ورب بدهن المشيرج
الطري المغسول والسكر الابيض ومتى خلط في ماكول شرب
عليه الماء الحار والسكنجبين واستطفه بالقي فان كانت الطبيعة
يابسه اتبع الجلنجبين على الزنجبيل واكل الماء حمص بدهن الشيرج
المغسول فان كانت الطبيعه معتدله اكل الخل والزيت الموصوف
قبل الباب الثالث في الحمى التي تنوب غبا
وهي الصفراوية هذه الحمى تتولد من الصفرا العفنة اذا غلبت
على الكبد والعروق وينبغي في علاجها اذا كانت خالصة ولم
يكن صاحبها شرهما ماء الشعير والسكنجبين الساذج واكل
الخبز المغسول بماء الرمان الحامض وماء الحصرم فان كانت الطبيعه
يابسه فشراب الاجاص والمزورات المتخذة من الاسفاناخ
والقرع ودهن اللوز الباب الرابع
في الحمى التي تنوب يوما ويومين وهي السوداوية هذه الحمى
تتولد من السودا العفنة اذا غلبت على الطحال وساير العروق
وينبغي في علاجها اذا كانت خالصه والعليل شره ان يسقى ايام

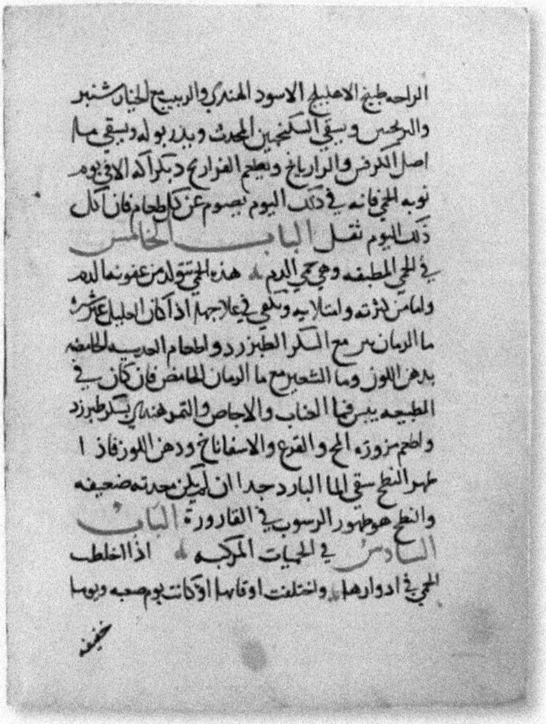

الراحه طبخ الاهليلج الاسود الهندي والربيع لخيار شنبر
والترنجبين ويسقي السكنجبين المحدث ويذر بوله ويسقي ما
اصل الكرفس والرازيانج ويطعم الفراريج ويكرر ذلك الا في يوم
نوبه الحمي فانه في ذلك اليوم يصوم عن كل طعام فان اكل
ذلك اليوم ثقل الباب الخامس
في الحمي المطبقه وهي حمي الدم هذه الحمي تتولد من عفونه الدم
ولما من كثرته وامتلايه ويكفي في علاجه اذا كان الحليل عشره
ما الرمان مع السكر الطبرزد والطعام الحريره الحامضه
بدهن اللوز وما الشعير مع ما الرمان الحامض فان كان في
الطبيعه يبس فيها الخباب والاجاص والتمر هندي بسكر طبرزد
والطعم مزوره الحب والقرع والاسفاناخ ودهن اللوز فاذا
ظهر النضج سقي الما البارد جدا ان لم يكن معدته ضعيفه
والنضج هو ظهور الرسوب في القارورة الباب
السادس في الحميات المركبه اذا اختلط
الحمي في ادوارها واختلفت اوقاتها او كانت يوم صعبه ويوما

تخفف

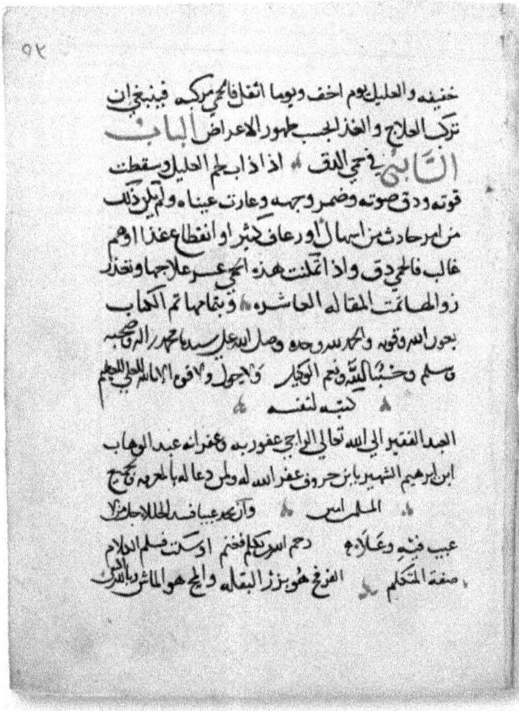

٩٢

خفيفه والعليل يوم اخف ويوما اثقل فالحمي مركبه فينبغي ان
ترك العلاج والغذ لحسب ظهور الاعراض الباب
الثاني في حمي الدق • اذا ذاب لحم العليل وسقطت
قوته ودق صوته وضمر وجهه وغارت عيناه ولم يكن ذلك
من امر حادث من اسهال او رعاف كثير او انقطاع غذا او هم
غالب فالحمي دق واذا اتمكنت هذه الحمي عسر علاجها وتعذر
زوالها تمت المقاله العاشره • وبتمامها تم الكتاب
بعون الله وقوته والحمد لله وحده وصلى الله على سيدنا محمد والرضى صحبه
وسلم وحسبنا الله ونعم الوكيل ولا حول ولا قوة الا بالله العلي العظيم
• كتبه لنفسه •
العبد الفقير الي الله تعالى الراجي عفو ربه وغفرانه عبد الوهاب
ابن ابرهيم الشهير بابن حروف غفر الله له ولمن دعا له بالمغفرة آمين
• المسلمين • وان تجد عيبا فسد الخللا جل من لا
عيب فيه وعلا • رحم الله امرئ تكلم فغنم او سكت فسلم الكلام
صفة المتكلم • الفرغ هو بزر البقله والحج هو الماش بالفارسية